Foreword

It all began with a "Wicker" tote bag.

Tamara first contacted me to buy some of our Platypus Designer Duct Tape in May of 2011. I am the product designer of this brand of duct tape and own the company that sells it.

Shortly after buying quite a few rolls she wrote to tell me that our "Wicker" patterned tape was her new favorite. One of the reasons I started the Platypus line was to foster creativity, and hearing testaments like this from our customers makes me happy.

Tamara also attached a photo of a tote that she'd made with the "Wicker" Designer Duct Tape. When I opened the file, it seemed as if everything stopped. People use our tape for many things, and I'd seen quite a few examples of crafts, but I'd never seen anything on this level. Her design was stylish, unexpected, and crafted with a high-level of precision. It was simply stunning when compared to all the other crafts I'd seen. I immediately contacted her. We hit it off right away and began collaborating. I asked her to design and create a number of projects for us.

These projects for my company included a "Modern Houndstooth" bejeweled clutch, a "Blue Paisley" and "Argyle" wedding bouquet with matching "Blue Paisley" cummerbund and bow tie, a "Platypus Orange Linen" and "White Linen" shoulder bag, "Pink Polka Dot" snow boots, and more. I think her designs should be sold in chic boutiques. She's that good.

I anxiously awaited her packages, knowing that the projects held within would surpass my expectations. I went around the office showing the projects, saying, "Look! Check this out! Isn't this amazing?!"

Tamara has a keen eye for color and pattern and a knack for manipulating duct tape. She works like both a fashion designer and a seamstress, creating templates for her designs and planning each step carefully.

She is great at interpreting ideas and making them her own. For photo or film shoots, my team often gave her inspirational imagery and color combinations for props. Tamara took creative direction incredibly professionally and delivered top-notch work. Once we were in a serious time crunch to make a whole slew of gift box bows, letters, and flowers to appear within a Christmas scene composed of Platypus Designer Duct Tape. Despite how busy she was, Tamara rose to the challenge and delivered dozens of beautiful crafts on time, flawlessly. Everything looked amazing on camera.

It is my hope that Tamara's creativity shown within this book inspires your own, and that your life will become more beautiful—and more fun—by crafting with duct tape.

Sincerely,
Rob Jordan
Owner | Product Designer
Platypus Designer Duct Tape™
Designerducttape.com

Dazzling Duct Tape Designs

Fashionable Accessories, Adorable Décor and Many More Creative Crafts You Make at Home

Tamara Boykins

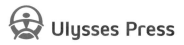

Published in the U.S. by
Ulysses Press
P.O. Box 3440
Berkeley, CA 94703
www.ulyssespress.com

ISBN: 978-1-61243-133-8
Library of Congress Control Number 2012951889

Printed in the United States by Bang Printing

10 9 8 7 6 5 4 3 2

Acquisitions Editor: Kelly Reed
Managing Editor: Claire Chun
Editor: Lauren Harrison
Proofreader: Elyce Berrigan-Dunlop
Design and layout: what!design @ whatweb.com
Production: Jake Flaherty
Photographs: Tamara Boykins except rolled out blue duct tape © Lasse Kristensen/
    shutterstock.com, duct tape on page iii and in page folio © caliber_3D/shutterstock.com

Distributed by Publishers Group West

Table of Contents

Introduction

Duct tape isn't just for repairs anymore. It has come out of the toolbox and is now used to create purses, jewelry, home décor, and even clothing. It comes in dozens of brilliant colors and patterns and is a fun and inexpensive way to express creativity. Duct tape crafts are durable and not messy, which makes them the perfect pastime for individuals, parties, classrooms, and rainy days.

My love of creating with duct tape began when one of my sons went shopping for a new wallet but couldn't find one that he liked. I picked up a few rolls to try to make him one and haven't put them down yet. With a little duct tape and lots of imagination, the possibilities for hours of entertainment are endless.

Getting Started

These primary supplies will help you create all of your designs. Projects that require additional materials will include a list on their page.

■ ■ ■ ■ ■ ■ ■ ■ ■ ■ ■ ■ ■

WHAT YOU'LL NEED

Duct tape rolls
Scissors
Cutting mat
Hard, flat surface
Craft knife
Ruler
Pen

■ ■ ■ ■ ■ ■ ■ ■ ■ ■ ■ ■ ■

TAMARA'S TIPS

Here are a few useful tips I've figured out along the way through much trial and error.

■ A self-healing cutting mat is ideal. Not only does it protect your surface but it has dimensions printed right on it, making measuring a breeze.

■ Nonstick scissors are terrific for cutting supersticky duct tape. It's also possible to tear tape by hand by holding each side firmly and pulling them quickly in opposite directions.

■ Craft knives can be quick and easy for cutting slits and angles but are very sharp. They should be used with caution and under adult supervision.

■ Layering is a great way to make your projects sturdy and durable. To avoid flimsy projects, try adding a second or third layer of tape.

■ Use gray duct tape for layering and areas that aren't readily seen. Gray comes in larger rolls and is cheaper per inch than patterns and colors. Make your patterned tape rolls last longer by lining your projects with gray.

■ Cut tape pieces a little longer than you'll need them for your finished project to allow room for accurate trimming.

■ Always press and smooth tape strips with your fingers to make sure they're adhered and flat.

■ Corner wrapping and angle trimming are both great ways to avoid loose, sticky edges. Both methods will be explained.

■ A heavy duty or leather hole punch works best on thick, layered duct tape.

■ The best way to reinforce a hole is by using an eyelet.

■ Using self-stick gems, foam letters, and other decorations is a great way to personalize your creations.

TECHNIQUES

DOUBLE-SIDED STRIP

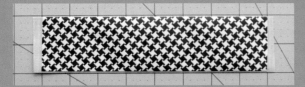

Unroll and measure a strip of tape. Cut it to the desired length and lay it sticky-side up on your cutting mat. Cut another strip of tape the same length and place it directly on top of the first strip so that the sticky sides meet.

STRIP WITH STICKY OVERHANG

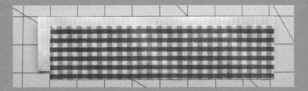

Begin constructing a double-sided tape strip, but instead of placing the strip directly on top, place it ¼ inch below the long edge, leaving exposed adhesive.

SINGLE-SIDED FABRIC SHEET

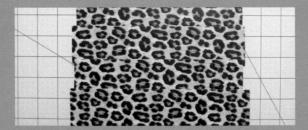

Cut a strip of tape to the desired length and lay it sticky-side down on your cutting mat.

Cut another strip of the same length and place it sticky-side down on top of the first strip overlapping it at least ¼ inch. Repeat until you have achieved the sheet size that you need, and trim the ends to their finished size.

DOUBLE-SIDED FABRIC SHEET

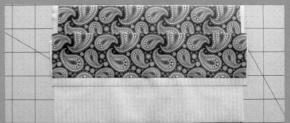

Create a single-sided fabric sheet in the desired size. Peel it up and flip it over so that the sticky side is facing up. Cut additional strips of tape the same length. Starting at the edge, lay a strip on top so that the sticky sides meet. Continue to overlap strips until you have reached the other edge and all adhesive is covered, and trim the ends to their finished size.

DOUBLE-SIDED FABRIC SHEET WITH OVERHANG ON ALL FOUR SIDES

Create a single-sided fabric sheet and trim the ends to their finished size.

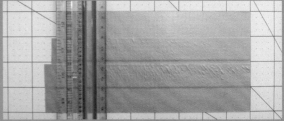

Cut the strips for the second side that are 2 inches longer than the first side. Center the first strip 1 inch above the top edge, leaving 1 inch of exposed adhesive on the top and both ends. Repeat on the bottom edge.

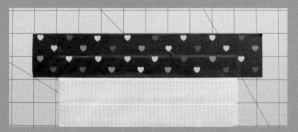

Fill in the middle by overlapping strips until you reach the center and all adhesive is covered.

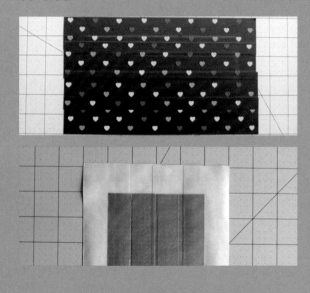

DOUBLE-SIDED FABRIC SHEET WITH OVERHANG ON THREE SIDES

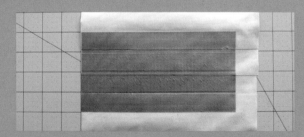

Create a double-sided fabric sheet with four overhangs and trim off one short side.

DOUBLE-SIDED FABRIC SHEET WITH OVERHANG ON TWO SIDES

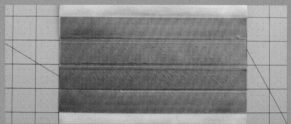

Create a double-sided fabric sheet with four overhangs and trim off two opposite short sides.

SINGLE-LAYER FOLDED STRAP

Measure and cut a strip of tape to the desired length and place it sticky-side up on your cutting mat. Fold one side in toward the center almost halfway and press down firmly.

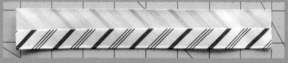

Turn your tape strip around and fold the other side over, covering the first. Be sure not to fold past the edge of the first fold.

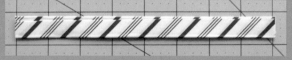

DOUBLE-LAYER FOLDED STRAP

Create a single-layer folded strap. Cut a second strip of tape the same length and place it sticky side up.

Lay the first strap down in the center of the sticky side.

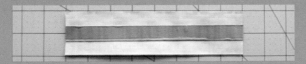

Fold in the sides to cover the original strap.

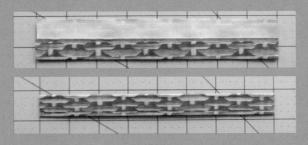

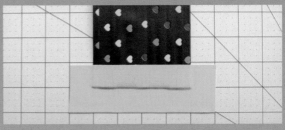

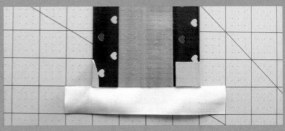

Flip the project over. Cut a slit on the side that is even with the edge of your project and fold in. Repeat on the other end.

TRIMMING EDGES

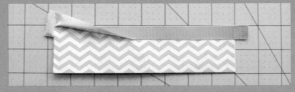

Cut a strip of tape slightly longer than the edge you need to cover. Place the strip of tape halfway over one side of the edge. Flip the project over and fold the remaining tape down on the other side and trim the excess tape.

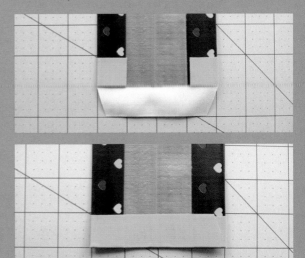

Make angled cuts from the corners of your project to the ends of the overhang and fold in the flap.

WRAPPING CORNERS

One great way to avoid loose, sticky edges is to wrap your corners.

Begin with a strip that is at least 1 inch longer than your project on both sides. Place the strip halfway over the edge of the finished side.

Around the House

Including handmade items in the décor of your home can help add originality and character to your spaces. Whether made out of duct tape or other materials, items created by my children or me can be found in every room of our house.

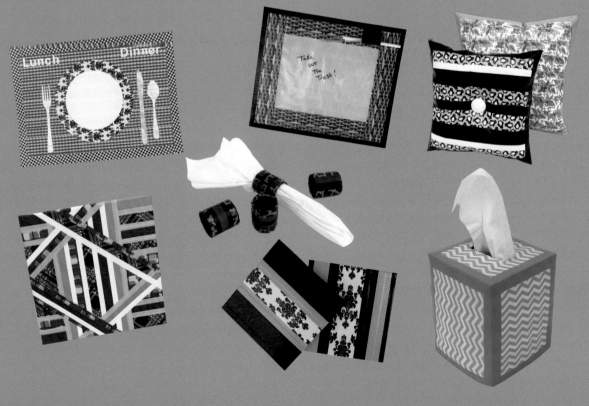

Coasters

Protect your surfaces with custom coasters. Your guests will be amazed when you hand them one of these to set their drinks on.

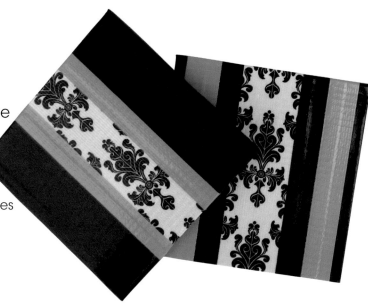

■ ■ ■ ■ ■ ■ ■ ■ ■ ■ ■

ADDITIONAL MATERIALS:

Cardboard, wood squares, or square tiles
Sheet of cork
Glue for plastics or hot glue gun
Clear duct tape (optional)

■ ■ ■ ■ ■ ■ ■ ■ ■ ■ ■

1 To use cardboard, cut out a 4¼-inch square. If the cardboard is thin, glue two squares together.

2 Create a 10-inch square single-sided fabric sheet (page ix).

3 Cover the finished, nonsticky side of the sheet with clear duct tape, if desired.

4 Place your fabric sheet sticky-side up and place the cardboard, wood, or tile in the center.

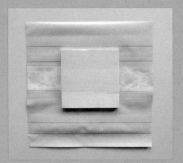

5 On one side, cut slits even with the ends of the cardboard, wood, or tile and fold in the flap that's created.

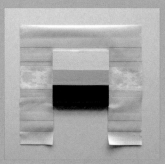

6 Repeat on the other three sides.

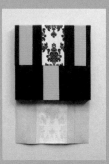

7 Cut a 4-inch square of cork and attach it to the bottom of the coaster with glue.

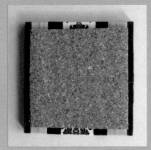

8 Use small pieces of clear duct tape on the corners to keep them from lifting.

Napkin Rings

Use your favorite duct tape patterns to add an unexpected finishing touch to your table.

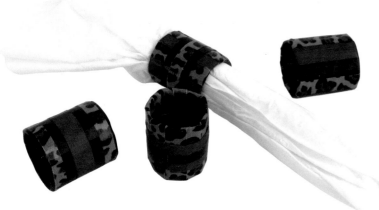

1 Create a 12 x 1¼-inch double-sided strip (page ix).

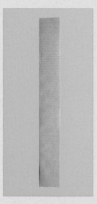

2 Make a cylinder out of the strip by rolling it up to the size you want for your napkin ring and securing it with a piece of tape.

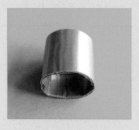

3 Cut many ½ x 3¼-inch strips of tape to cover the roll.

4 Lay the strips evenly across the roll and tuck the ends on the inside. Be sure to overlap the strips slightly.

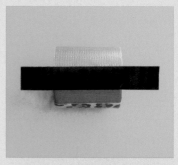

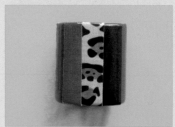

Reversible Placemats

Cook up some mealtime excitement by making placemats that will also keep things tidy.

■ ■ ■ ■ ■ ■ ■ ■ ■ ■ ■

ADDITIONAL MATERIALS:

Dishes and utensils for tracing
Clear duct tape

■ ■ ■ ■ ■ ■ ■ ■ ■ ■ ■

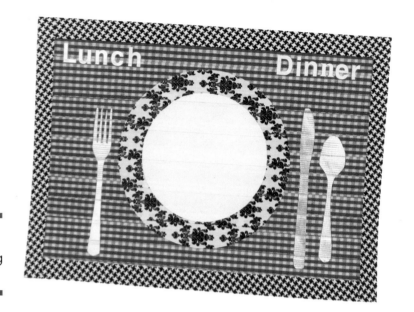

1 Create a 13 x 18-inch double-sided fabric sheet (page ix). Use a different color on each side for a unique reversible mat.

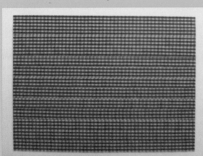

2 Cut two 18-inch strips and two 13-inch strips in half lengthwise and use the strips to create a border around the placemat.

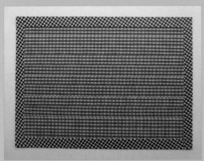

3 Create a single-sided fabric sheet that is slightly larger than the plate you intend to trace (page ix).

4 Trace the plate onto the single-sided sheet, cut it out, and stick it to the placemat wherever you like.

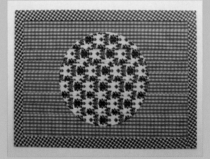

5 To create a smaller circle in the center of the plate, trace and cut out a smaller plate or bowl. Create more single-sided fabric sheets as needed.

6 Trace and cut out shapes for utensils and a cup, if desired.

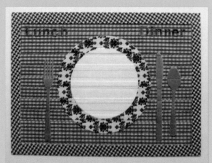

7 Cover the placemat with clear duct tape for easier cleanup.

8 Repeat on the other side of the placemat with the same or a different design.

9 To create an adorable pet mat, follow the same steps to construct the mat and decorate by tracing and cutting out circles to represent the food and water bowls.

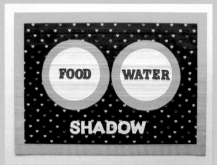

Decorative Pillow

Whether on a sofa, chair, or bed, a duct tape pillow will definitely make a statement.

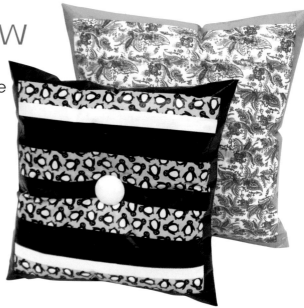

▪ ▪ ▪ ▪ ▪ ▪ ▪ ▪ ▪ ▪ ▪ ▪ ▪

ADDITIONAL MATERIALS:
Fiber fill or batting

OPTIONAL SUPPLIES:
Two buttons
Large needle
Thick thread or string

▪ ▪ ▪ ▪ ▪ ▪ ▪ ▪ ▪ ▪ ▪ ▪ ▪

1 Create two 12-inch square double-sided fabric sheets (page ix).

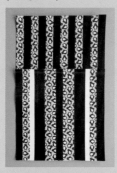

2 Stack the sheets together with the wrong sides facing out.

3 Trim three of the edges with 12-inch strips of tape to secure the sides together (page xi).

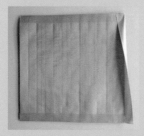

4 Turn the pillow right-side out and trim the same three sides with 12-inch strips of tape.

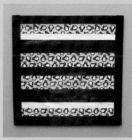

5 Fill the pillow through the open end and seal shut with a 12-inch strip of tape.

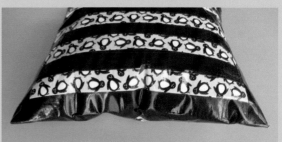

ADDING BUTTONS:

1 Mark the center of the pillow on both sides.

2 Cut a long piece of thread and fold it in half.

3 Thread the folded end of the string through the hole in one of the buttons.

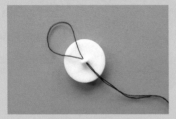

4 Thread the open ends into the loop and pull through.

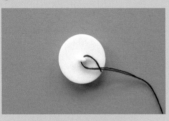

5 Thread the open ends into the eye of the needle.

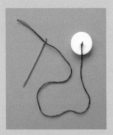

6 Carefully insert the needle into the center of the pillow and push it out the center of the other side.

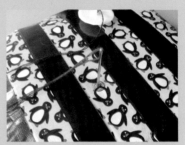

7 Pull the string all the way out and remove the needle.

8 Thread one of the open ends of the string through the hole in the other button.

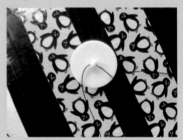

9 Tie one loop in the string (just like the first step in tying your shoes) and pull the buttons in as tight as you want.

10 Make several knots to secure the button, then trim the excess string.

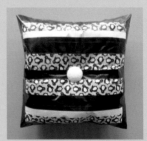

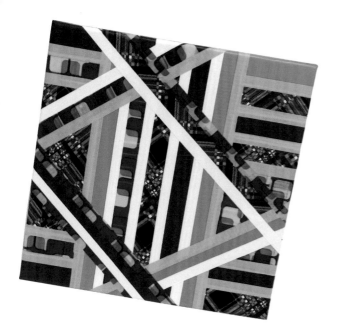

Canvas Art

Finding the perfect pictures to complement a space can be difficult. So stop looking and make some!

■ ■ ■ ■ ■ ■ ■ ■ ■ ■ ■ ■ ■ ■

ADDITIONAL MATERIALS:
Framed canvas
Pencil

■ ■ ■ ■ ■ ■ ■ ■ ■ ■ ■ ■ ■ ■

1 Sketch the design you would like to create on the canvas.

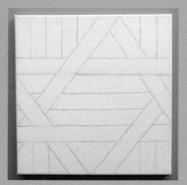

2 Cut strips of tape in the sizes needed to fill in the pattern.

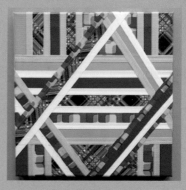

Tissue Box Cover

Dress up those boring store-bought tissue boxes with duct tape covers that match your room and your personality.

■ ■ ■ ■ ■ ■ ■ ■ ■ ■ ■ ■ ■

ADDITIONAL MATERIALS:

Square box of tissues

■ ■ ■ ■ ■ ■ ■ ■ ■ ■ ■ ■ ■

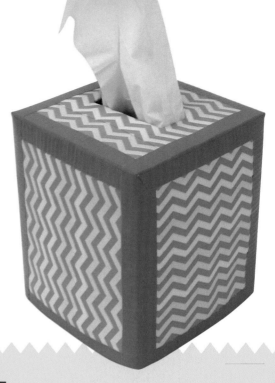

1 Create four 4½ x 5¼-inch double-sided fabric sheets and one 4½-inch square double-sided sheet (page ix).

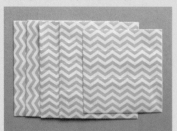

2 In the center of the 4½-inch square sheet, measure and draw a 1 x 2½-inch rectangle.

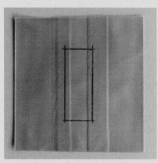

3 Draw a 1½-inch line lengthwise down the center of the rectangle, then finish the line on each end with a triangle that connects at the corners.

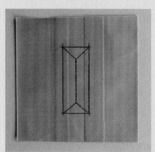

4 Cut on the center line and the triangles to form an opening.

5 Fold back the four flaps you've created and use strips of tape to secure them in place.

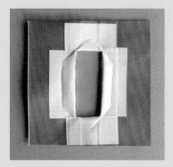

6 To assemble the sides, arrange the remaining sheets on the cutting mat with the wrong sides up. The square should be in the center with the four rectangles on the sides.

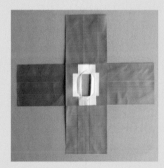

7 Cut two 4½-inch strips of tape in half lengthwise and use them to attach the four sides to the square.

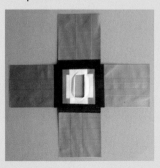

8 Cut four 5¼-inch strips and place them halfway over each side of two opposite rectangles.

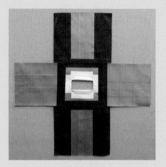

9 Lift a side with overhang and the side next to it. With the overhang on the inside, line the edges up and connect them to create a corner. Be sure to press down the tape on the inside.

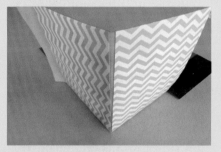

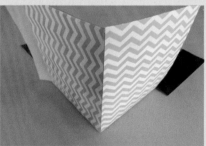

10 Repeat with the other sides and turn the cover over.

11 Cut a 4½-inch strip of tape in half lengthwise and use the strips to cover the top seams on two opposite sides.

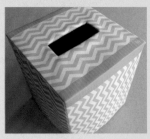

12 Cut two additional 4½-inch strips of tape in half lengthwise and use them to trim the four bottom edges (page xi).

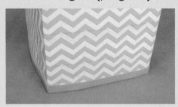

13 Now cut a 16-inch strip of tape in half lengthwise. On one of the remaining sides, center the strip over the top seam and bring it down around either side.

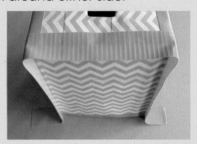

14 Cut a slit in the top corners and lay the tape flat.

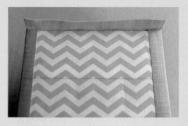

15 Fold the remaining tape around the bottom to the inside.

16 Repeat on the other side.

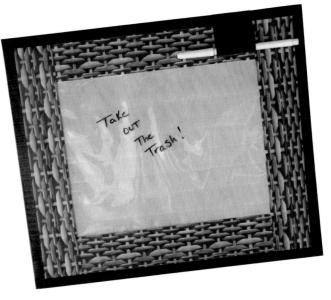

Dry Erase Board

∎ ∎ ∎ ∎ ∎ ∎ ∎ ∎ ∎ ∎ ∎

ADDITIONAL MATERIALS:
Sheet protector
Adhesive-backed magnets
Dry erase marker

∎ ∎ ∎ ∎ ∎ ∎ ∎ ∎ ∎ ∎ ∎

1 To begin the board, cut the strip of holes off the sheet protector.

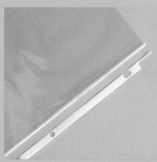

2 Create an 8½ x 11-inch double-sided fabric sheet (page ix) and slide it into the protector.

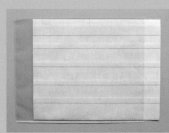

3 Create a 13 x 15-inch single-sided fabric sheet and lay it sticky-side up (page ix).

4 Center the sheet protector on the single-sided sheet and adhere it with the finished side (the side you'll write on) up.

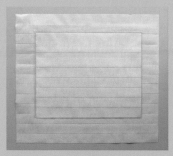

5 Cut enough 13-inch strips of tape to cover the exposed adhesive on the shorter ends and 15-inch strips to cover the longer sides. Be sure to overlap the tape onto the sheet protector on all four sides to secure it.

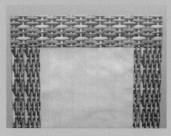

6 Cut two 15-inch strips of tape to trim the 15-inch sides and two additional 15-inch strips to wrap the 13-inch ends (page xi).

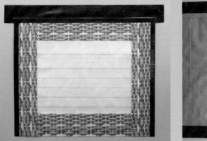
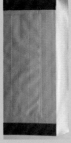

7 Add magnets to the back of the board.

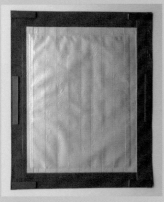

8 To add a marker holder, create a 10-inch double-sided strip (page ix) and place it across the marker.

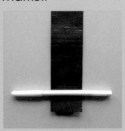

9 Fold up the end of the strip to create a loop around the marker.

10 Use a 1 x 4-inch strip of tape to secure the loop. Fold the ends around the back.

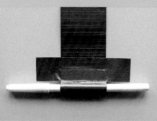

11 Place the strip with the marker near the top of the board where desired and secure to the front with a small strip of tape.

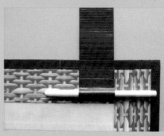

12 Fold the remainder of the strip over the top of the board and secure on the back with several strips of tape.

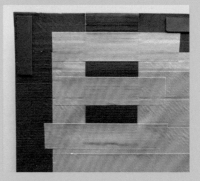

All Things Girly

All of the girls I know love craft projects, especially the wearable kind. There are so many colorful duct tape patterns available today that it's easy to bring crafting and fashion together and create these stylish accessories.

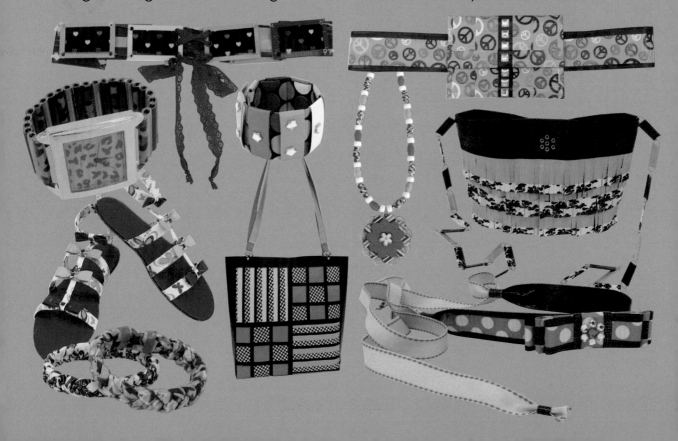

Braided Bangle

A girl can never have too many bangles. Create your own look by mixing and matching different colors and patterns.

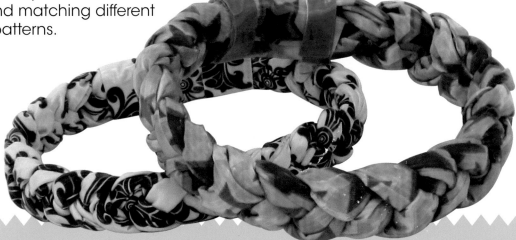

1 Create three 14-inch single-layer folded straps (page x). For a thicker bracelet, make double-layer straps.

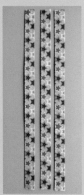

2 Braid the strands together as tightly as possible. When working alone, a clipboard works great to hold the ends of the strips.

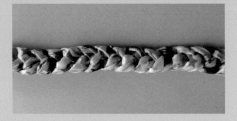

3 Wrap small strips of tape around each end to keep them from unraveling.

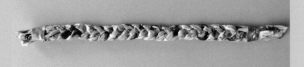

4 Determine how long you need the bracelet to be so that it will slip on and off comfortably, and cut the ends accordingly. Make sure there's tape wrapped around the area you are going to cut so the ends don't unravel.

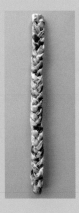

5 Place the flat ends of the bracelet together. Center a 4-inch strip of tape over both ends of the bracelet and wrap it around to seal them together.

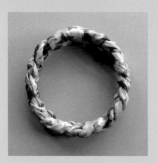

6 If you want, use small strips of tape to cover the seams.

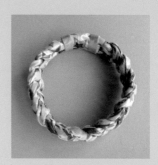

3D Cuff

Stir up excitement with this cuff-style bracelet that literally pops off your wrist.

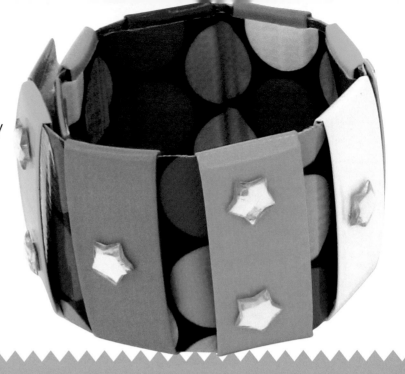

■ ■ ■ ■ ■ ■ ■ ■ ■ ■ ■ ■ ■

ADDITIONAL MATERIALS:
Velcro

■ ■ ■ ■ ■ ■ ■ ■ ■ ■ ■ ■ ■

1 Create a double-sided strip that's at least 2 inches longer than your wrist size (page ix).

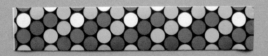

2 Trim the strip down so that it's 1½ inches wide.

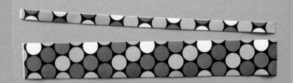

3 Create several 3½-inch single-layer folded straps (page x). The number of straps you'll need depends on the size of your wrist.

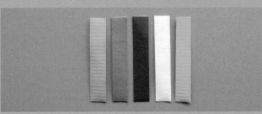

4 Place a single-layer folded strap across the strip. Fold the ends around the back and secure with a piece of tape.

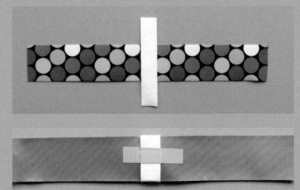

5 Add as many straps as desired. Be sure to leave enough room for the fastener.

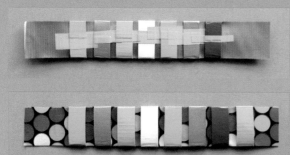

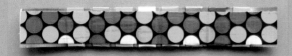

6 Cut a strip of tape to cover the inside of the bracelet then trim off any excess length.

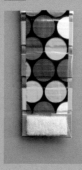

7 Wrap the ends (page xi).

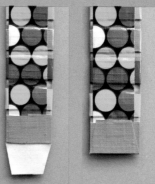

8 Add the Velcro.

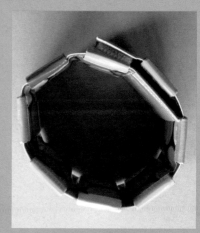

Headband

Headbands are a fun way to accessorize. Make one to match every outfit and wear a new one every day.

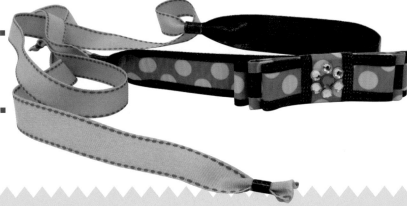

ADDITIONAL MATERIALS:

Ribbon
Stapler

1 To make the headband, create a 14-inch double-sided strip and cut it in half lengthwise (page ix).

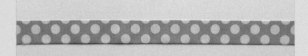

2 Use a 14-inch strip of tape cut in half lengthwise to trim each edge (page xi).

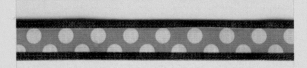

3 Create three more double-sided strips that are 6, 7, and 8 inches long. Cut them in half lengthwise.
Tip: Use the remaining half of the 14-inch strip for a coordinated look.

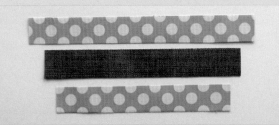

4 Use three additional strips of tape in the same three lengths, cut in half lengthwise to trim each double-sided strip.

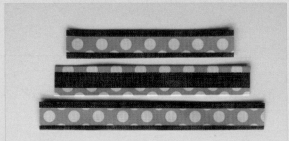

5 Place the three strips wrong-side up on the cutting mat. Fold in the ends so that they meet in the center and secure with a piece of tape.

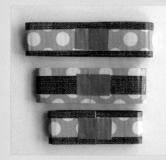

6 Stack the folded strips largest to smallest, and place them on the headband where desired.

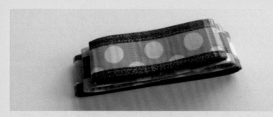

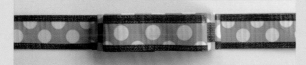

7 Cut a 4-inch strip of tape in half lengthwise and wrap it around the strips and the headband to join them together.

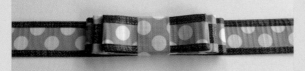

8 Use two smaller strips to cover the seams.

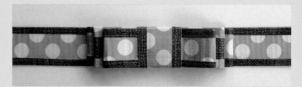

9 Staple a piece of ribbon to the end of the headband.

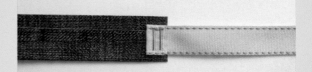

10 Carefully fold the end in half and secure it with a small strip of tape.

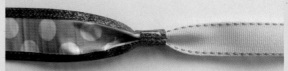

11 Repeat on the other end and trim the ribbon to the desired length.

12 Use small strips of tape to secure the ribbon at the ends.

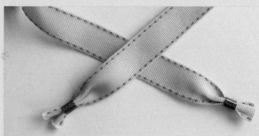

Beaded Necklace with Matching Pendant

Everyone will ask where you got such a delightful necklace because they won't be able to find beads like these in any store.

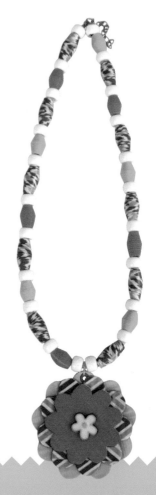

■ ■ ■ ■ ■ ■ ■ ■ ■ ■ ■ ■

ADDITIONAL MATERIALS:

Ruler
Drinking straws
Thin necklace, ribbon, or yarn
Pony beads (optional)
Pendant Materials:
Hole punch
Eyelets (optional)
Single-loop button
Pipe cleaner
Thread

■ ■ ■ ■ ■ ■ ■ ■ ■ ■ ■ ■

1 To make the beads, cut a 10-inch strip of tape and place it sticky-side down on the cutting mat.

2 Place the ruler at the 1-inch mark on the cutting mat on one end, then angle the ruler to the corner of the other end.
Note: Make a line if needed, but it will show on the finished bead.

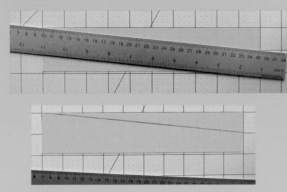

3 Cut off the angled strip of tape and place the end of it around a straw.

4 Roll the entire length of the strip around the straw.

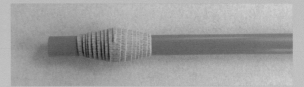

5 Trim the excess straw from both ends.

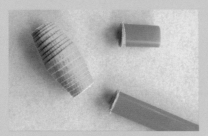

6 Use the same strip of tape to make additional beads by repeating the angle from the 1-inch mark on the other end. **Tip:** To make smaller beads, start with the ruler at the ¾ or ½-inch marks.

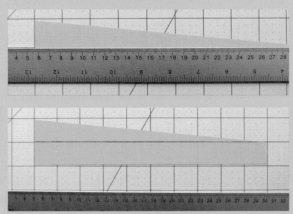

7 Make as many beads as desired and thread them onto the necklace, alternating with pony beads, if desired.

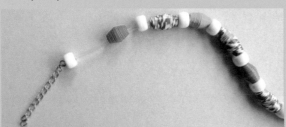

8 To make a pendant, cut any shape in various sizes out of double-sided fabric sheets (page ix).

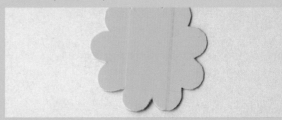

9 Make holes in the center of each shape. Insert eyelets into the holes, if using.

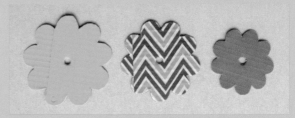

10 Stack the shapes from largest to smallest and place the button in the hole.

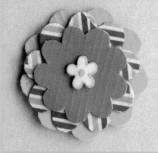

11 On the back, feed a pipe cleaner through the button hole; trim off the ends.

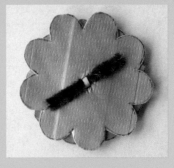

12 Cover and secure the pipe cleaner with strips of tape.

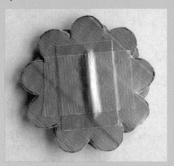

14 Tie the thread to the center of the necklace.

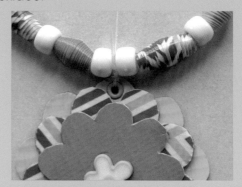

13 Make a hole in the largest shape for hanging. Tie a piece of thread through it.

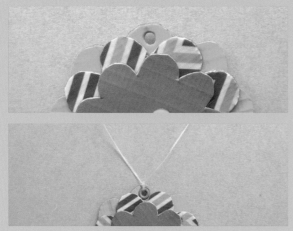

Waist Pouch

Not having pockets isn't a problem when you're sporting a custom-designed waist pouch that can carry small items.

ADDITIONAL MATERIALS:

Velcro

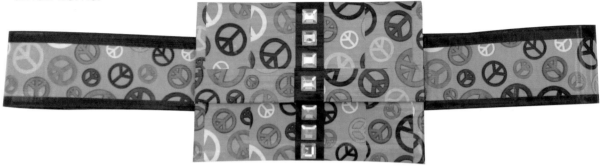

1 Begin the pouch by creating a 6 x 11-inch double-sided fabric sheet with overhang on three sides (page ix).

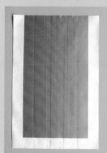

2 Cut slits in the overhang on the end that are even with the corners and fold in the flap created.

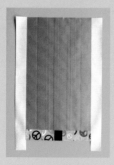

3 Measure 4 inches from the bottom of the folded end. Mark and cut slits in the overhang on both sides.

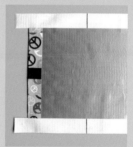

4 Fold in the flaps that are created on the sides of the unfinished end.

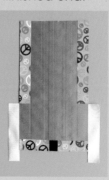

5 Cut angles in the corners of the remaining overhang.

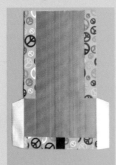

6 Between 5 and 8 inches from the folded bottom edge and 1½ inches from each side, mark and cut 2-inch lines to make slits for the belt.

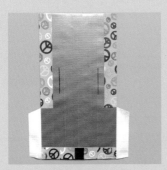

7 Create the pocket by folding the sheet at the 4-inch mark and using the overhang to secure the sides.

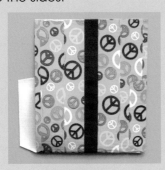

8 Cut an 8-inch strip of tape to wrap the unfinished end (page xi).

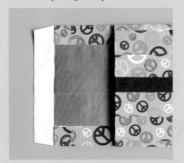

9 To make the belt, create a double-sided strip that's 2 inches longer than your waist (page ix).

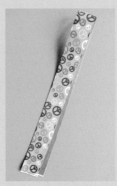

10 Cut two pieces of tape the same length as the strip and use them to trim both sides (page xi).

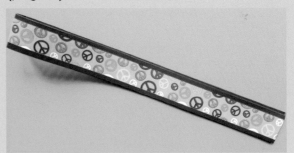

11 Connect the belt and pouch by sliding one end of the belt through the slits in the back of the pouch.

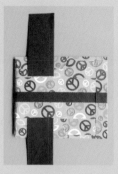

13 Cut two 4-inch pieces of tape and wrap both ends of the belt.

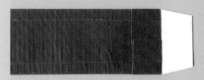

14 Add Velcro to the belt ends to fit.

12 Add Velcro to the pouch flap to secure it.

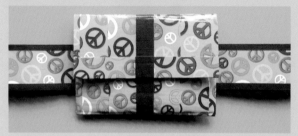

Laced Belt

What you wear can say a lot about you. Wearing a belt like this says that you're lots of fun.

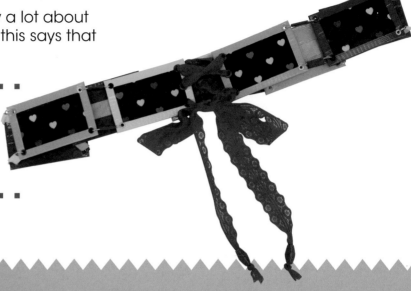

ADDITIONAL MATERIALS:

Hole punch
Eyelets (optional)
Paper clips
Ribbon or string

1 Create two 3-inch double-sided strips (page ix).

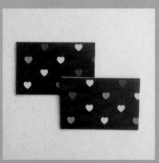

2 On each strip, use a 3-inch strip of tape cut in half lengthwise to trim the two sides (page xi).

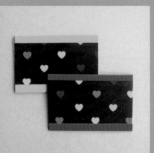

3 Use a 3½-inch strip cut in half lengthwise to wrap the ends (page xi).

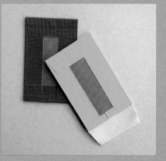

4 Punch a hole in each of the corners of both strips. Insert eyelets into the holes, if using.

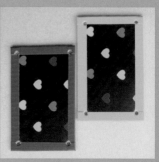

5 Place the open end of a paper clip through one of the holes on one strip and slide it around until it rests in the closed end.

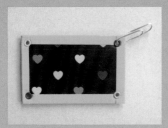

6 Repeat with the hole next to it.

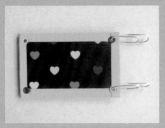

7 Slide the holes of the second strip onto the open end of the paper clips.

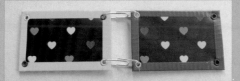

8 Cut strips of tape that are slightly smaller than the length of the paper clips and wrap them around each one.

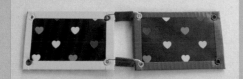

9 Continue to add paper clips and strips by repeating steps 1 to 8 until the belt is long enough to fit around your waist.

10 On the two end strips, make a third hole between the two corner holes.

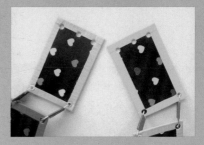

11 Lace a ribbon through the holes to create a closure for the belt.

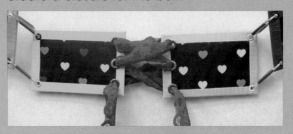

12 Thread duct tape beads (page 22) onto the ribbon and tie knots in the ends to secure.

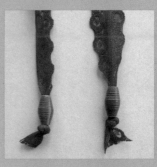

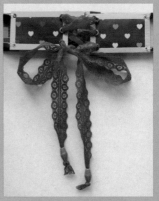

Stretchy Watchband

Watch bands should have their own personality just like you do. What kind will yours have?

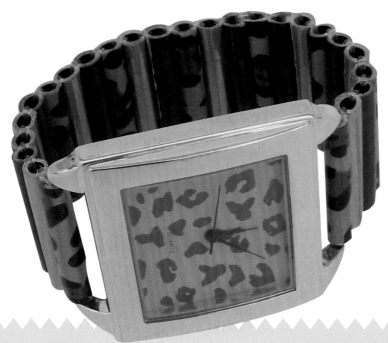

▪ ▪ ▪ ▪ ▪ ▪ ▪ ▪ ▪ ▪ ▪ ▪

ADDITIONAL MATERIALS:

Drinking straws
Watch face
Elastic jewelry cord

▪ ▪ ▪ ▪ ▪ ▪ ▪ ▪ ▪ ▪ ▪ ▪

1 Cut a strip of tape long enough to cover the straw.

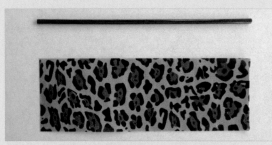

2 Roll the tape around the straw.

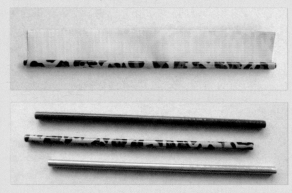

3 Cut pieces of wrapped straw the same length as the pin on the watch.

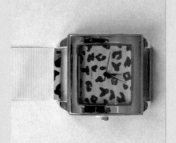

4 Cut a strip of tape to the width of the pin and wrap the end around the pin, leaving the adhesive exposed.

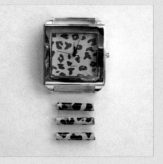

5 Cut a piece of elastic jewelry cord that is at least 48 inches long and center it against the pin.
Note: The length of cord needed may vary based on wrist size and the width of the watch.

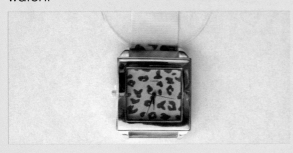

6 Wrap the tape around the cord and pin to join them.

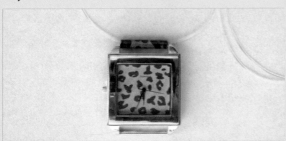

7 Place the ends of the cord through a straw piece in opposite directions and pull the cord tight.

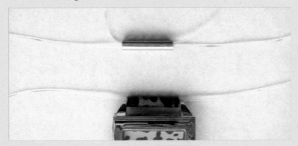

8 Continue threading wrapped straw pieces until there are enough to reach halfway around your wrist.

9 Temporarily tie off the end and begin the steps on the other side of the watch face.

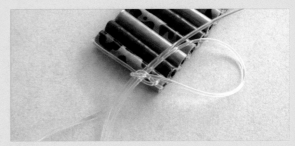

10 Once there are enough pieces to wrap comfortably around your wrist, join them by knotting together the cords and trimming the excess.

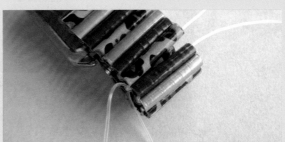

Fringed Sling

Have fun with fringe and carry your belongings in style. Crafty details make this cross-body bag a showstopper.

■ ■ ■ ■ ■ ■ ■ ■ ■ ■ ■

ADDITIONAL MATERIALS:

Velcro
Hole punch
Eyelets (optional)
Paper clips

■ ■ ■ ■ ■ ■ ■ ■ ■ ■ ■

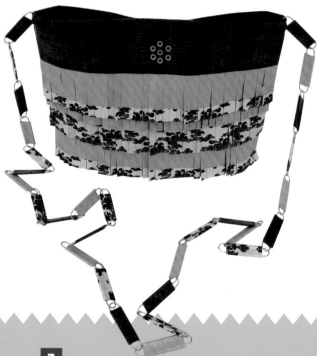

1 Create a 9 x 17-inch double-sided fabric sheet with overhang on both ends (page x).

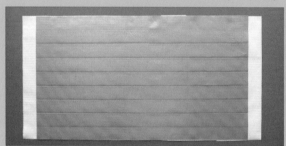

2 Fold in the overhang.

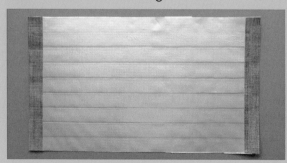

3 Fold the sheet in half and seal the sides together by trimming each one with a 9-inch strip of tape. Tuck the excess on the inside of the pouch.

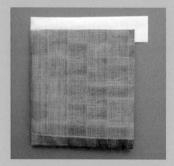

4 To make fringe, create a 3 x 9-inch single-sided fabric sheet (page ix) and place it sticky-side up on the cutting mat.

5 Create overhang by placing a 9-inch strip of tape on the sheet so that it hangs ¼ inch below the bottom edge.

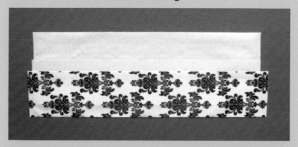

6 Place another 9-inch strip of tape on top, leaving at least ½ inch of adhesive exposed at the top.

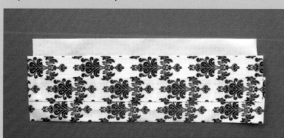

7 Flip the sheet over and fold up the ¼-inch of tape at the bottom. This will prevent the bottom edges of the fringe from being sticky.

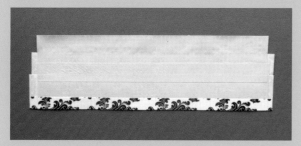

8 Cut slits along the length of the sheet without cutting into the exposed adhesive.

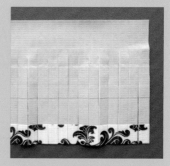

9 Attach the fringe to the bag 1 inch from the bottom edge.

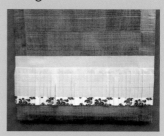

10 Place a 19-inch strip of tape around the entire bag to secure the fringe.

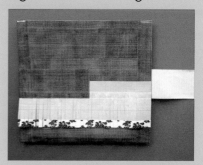

11 Continue making fringe and attaching it as desired.

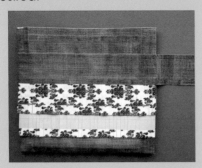

12 To give the bag a bottom, pinch together the bottom corners so they're flat.

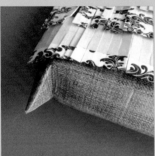

13 Fold the pinched corners toward the bottom of the bag and hold them in place with small pieces of tape.

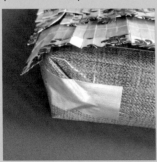

14 Cut two larger pieces of tape to conceal the folds.

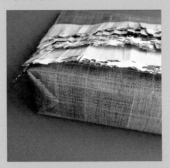

15 Add the Velcro to the inside center of the bag for closure.

16 Punch a hole near the top of both ends of the bag. Insert eyelets into the holes, if using.

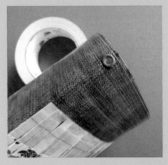

17 Create a strap by joining together enough paper clips to fit around your body.

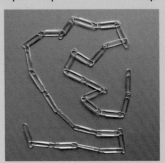

18 Cut strips of tape slightly smaller than the length of the paper clips to wrap around each one to secure it.

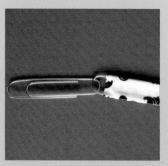

19 Be sure to insert the last two paper clips into the bag before wrapping them.

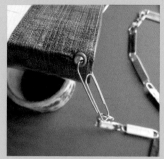

Four-Panel Tote

Since you have to carry your things in something, it might as well be in the cutest tote bag you've ever made.

■ ■ ■ ■ ■ ■ ■ ■ ■ ■ ■ ■ ■ ■

ADDITIONAL MATERIALS:

4 D-rings

■ ■ ■ ■ ■ ■ ■ ■ ■ ■ ■ ■ ■ ■

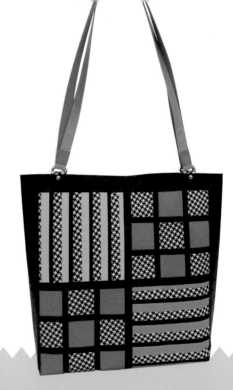

1 Create a 14 x 28-inch double-sided fabric sheet (page ix).

2 Leaving a 1-inch border around the outside, measure and draw two 12-inch squares, leaving 2 inches between them. Then divide the squares into four 6-inch squares.

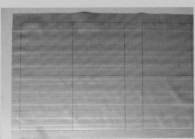

3 Create a design in each of the first four squares. In this case, I used overlapping straight lines and 2-inch squares in a checkerboard pattern. It's okay to extend the tape past the lines to the end, just remember that only the area inside the square will show.

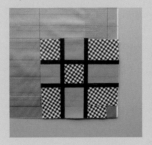
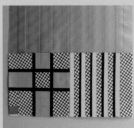

4 Use two narrow strips of tape to separate the four squares.

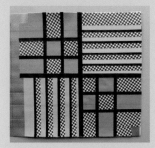

5 Repeat steps 3 and 4 with the four squares on the other side.

6 Use two 14-inch strips of tape to cover the 2-inch gap that separates the two halves.

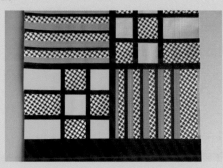

7 Cut two 28-inch and two 14-inch strips of tape and use them to trim the sides and ends of the sheet (page xi).

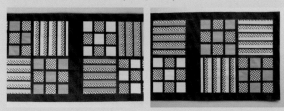

8 Flip the sheet over so the wrong side is facing up.

9 Create four 5-inch single-layer folded straps for attaching the handles (page x).

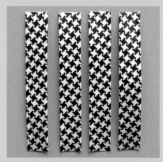

10 Slide each strap through a D-ring.

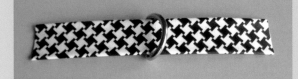

11 On one side of the sheet, position the ends of two straps where you want the handles be.

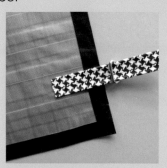

12 Secure the ends with a strip of tape.

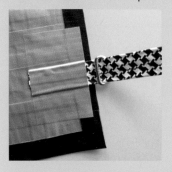

13 Fold down the other ends of the straps and secure them with several more strips of tape.

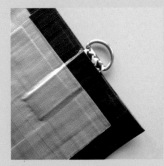

14 Repeat to attach the straps to the other end.

15 Fold the sheet in half and join the sides by trimming them with 15-inch strips of tape. Fold the excess down on the inside of the bag.

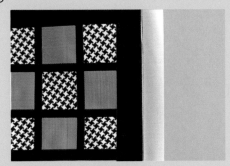

16 Pinch together about 2 inches of the bottom corners to create a flat bottom.

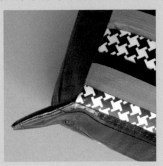

17 Fold the corner flaps toward the bottom or the side of the bag and use small pieces of tape to hold them in place.

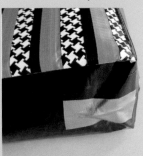

18 Cut two strips of tape that are at least 6 inches long and place one across each side and bottom of the bag to hide the flaps.

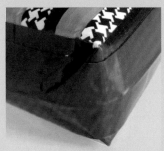

19 Create two 28-inch double-layer folded straps for handles (page x).

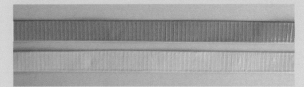

20 Place the end of a strap through a ring and fold it over about 1 inch.

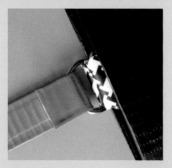

21 Cut a 6-inch strip of tape in half lengthwise and wrap it around the fold to secure it.

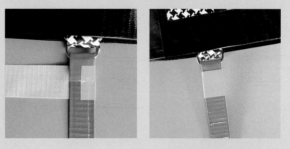

22 Repeat to finish attaching the handles.

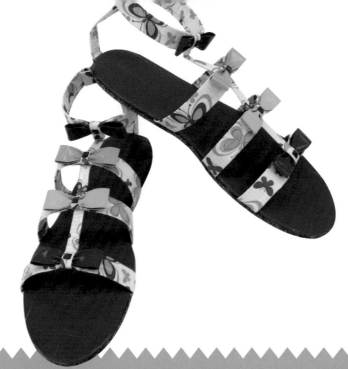

Bow Sandals

Mix and match your favorite patterns to design one-of-a-kind sandals to complement any outfit.

■ ■ ■ ■ ■ ■ ■ ■ ■ ■ ■ ■ ■ ■

ADDITIONAL MATERIALS:
Cardboard
Sheet of cork (optional)
Velcro
Hot glue gun or glue for plastics

■ ■ ■ ■ ■ ■ ■ ■ ■ ■ ■ ■ ■

1 Trace a pair of shoes or feet onto the cardboard and cut out the forms.

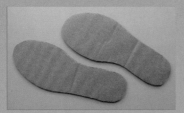

2 Trace and cut out the forms from cork as well. If cork is not available, a second layer of cardboard can be used.

3 Create a single-sided fabric sheet large enough to cover the cardboard form (page ix), and place the form in the center of the adhesive.

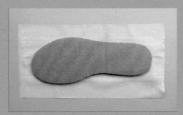

4 Cut slits around the outside of the form, creating small sections of tape. Fold them in toward the center.

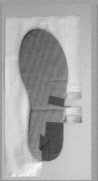
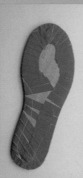
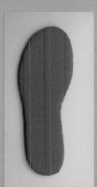

5 Create four double-layer folded straps that are at least 11 inches long and one that is 7 inches long (page x).

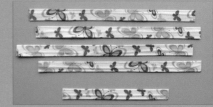

6 Create a very narrow double-layer folded strap that is also 11 inches long by cutting the strips of tape in half lengthwise before folding them (page x).

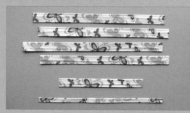

7 Create four 5-inch single-layer folded straps (page x).

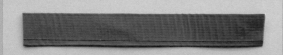

8 Fold in the ends of one 5-inch single-layer folded strap so that they meet in the center and secure with a small piece of tape.

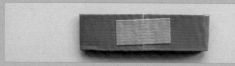

9 Center the folded strap on one of the 11-inch straps. Pinch the straps in the center to create a bow shape. Secure with a small strip of tape.

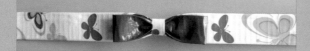

10 Repeat with the other three 5-inch straps.

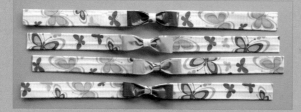

11 Take the narrow 11-inch strap and loop it around the center of the first bow. Secure it with a small strip of tape.

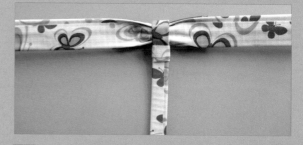

12 Add small tape strips to the back to reinforce.

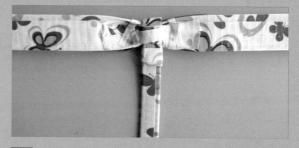

13 Based on the size of your foot, determine how far apart the next two straps should be and then secure them on the back with small strips of tape.

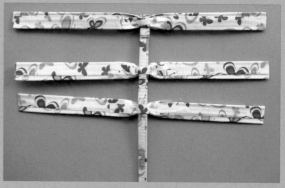

14 The remaining strap will be the ankle strap. Space it the same distance apart as the other two straps, and attach it the same as the first strap by creating a loop around the bow and securing it on the back with a strip of tape and several small strips.

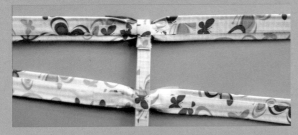

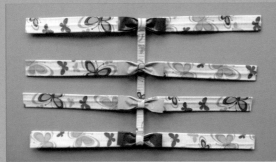

15 Secure the three foot straps to the cardboard form by trimming them as needed and taping them to the bottom of the form.

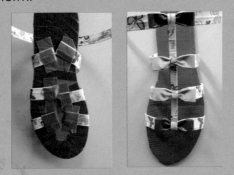

16 Trim and wrap the ends of the ankle strap (page xi).

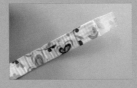

17 Tape the 7-inch strap to the bottom of the form at the center of the heel.

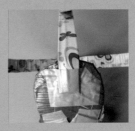

18 Loop the heel strap around the ankle strap and secure with a strip of tape.

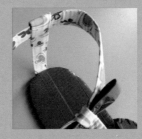

19 Add Velcro to fit.

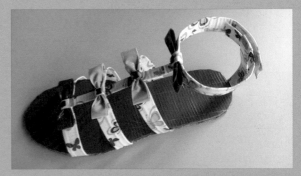

20 Glue the cork or second cardboard form to the bottom of the form.

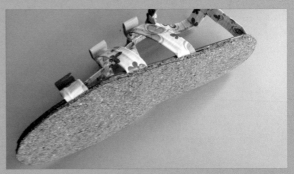

2 Cool 4 School

With so many people shopping at the same stores, it's almost impossible not to end up with the same school supplies as your classmates. That won't happen when you make some of your own out of duct tape.

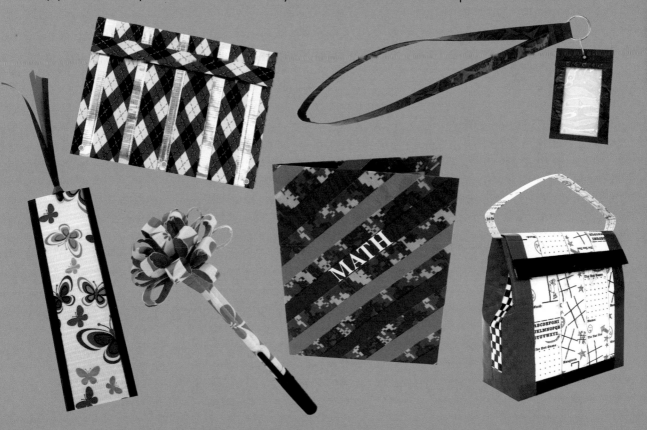

Bookmark

Reading is fundamental. Bookmarks made with your favorite duct tape patterns are just fun.

■ ■ ■ ■ ■ ■ ■ ■ ■ ■ ■ ■ ■ ■

ADDITIONAL MATERIALS:

Ribbon or yarn
Hole punch
Eyelet (optional)

■ ■ ■ ■ ■ ■ ■ ■ ■ ■ ■ ■ ■ ■

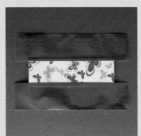

1 Create a 6-inch double-sided strip (page ix).

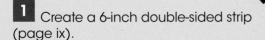

2 Cut an 8-inch strip of tape and place the tape evenly over the double-sided tape strip so that 1 inch of adhesive hangs over each end.

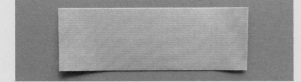

3 Turn the strip over and fold in the overhang.

4 Cut two additional 8-inch strips.

5 Place the strips ¼ to ½ inch over the edges of the finished side of the double-sided strip, then turn the bookmark over.

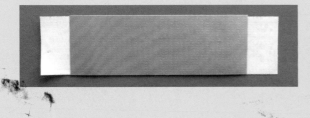
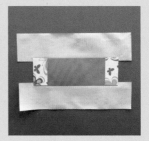

6 Wrap the corners (page xi).

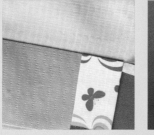 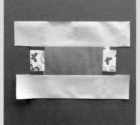

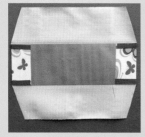 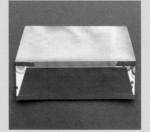

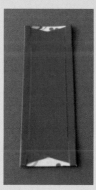 

7 Punch a hole just below the top edge. Insert an eyelet, if using.

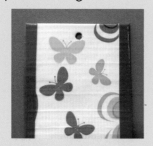

8 Add ribbon or yarn for fringe.

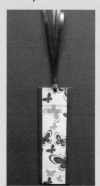

9 Cut angles in the corners, if desired.

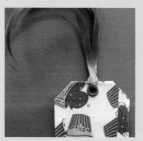

Lanyard with ID Holder

If you have to wear an ID badge daily, here's your chance to change your lanyard as often as you change your mind.

ADDITIONAL MATERIALS:

Split key ring
Lanyard hook
Badge holder
Hole punch
Eyelet (optional)

1 To make the lanyard, create a 32-inch double-layer strap (page x).

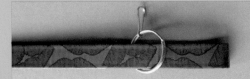

2 Slip the lanyard hook around the key ring, and slide the key ring onto the strap.

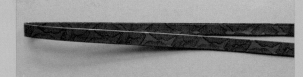

3 Before joining the ends, you need to create a twist so that the lanyard will lay flat against the body. Begin by folding the strap in half with the seam on the inside.

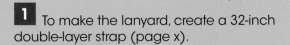

4 Flip over the end of the top strap so the seam is facing up. A twist should be formed.

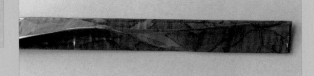

5 Keep the strap in this position and hold the flat ends of the strap together as if you were making a circle. Use a small piece of tape to help hold them in place.

6 Wrap a 3-inch strip of tape evenly around the ends to connect them. Make sure that you are joining one finished end and one with the seam showing.

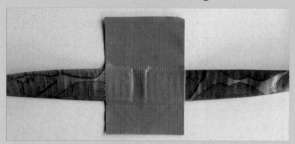

7 Bring your key ring with hook down into the sealed fold.

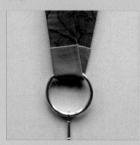

8 Form a V shape with the sealed ends and wrap the seam with a 3½ x ⅓-inch strip of tape. Add another thin strip of tape to finish.

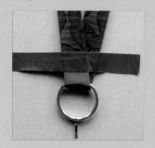
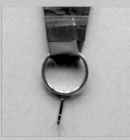

9 To create a matching holder, trim the sides of a badge holder with two small strips of tape (page xi). Be sure not to seal the opening.

10 Wrap the top and bottom of the holder, still being careful not to seal the opening (page xi).

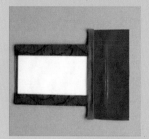
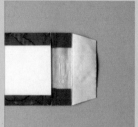

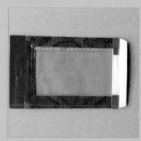

11 Make a new hole where the existing hole was. Insert an eyelet, if using.

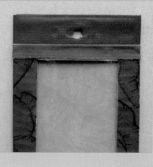

Folder

No one else in school will have folders like this. Make one for every subject.

- - - - - - - - - - - -

ADDITIONAL MATERIALS:

Hole punch (optional)

- - - - - - - - - - - -

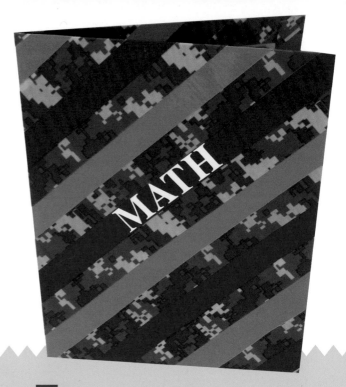

1 Create a 16 x 19-inch double-sided sheet with overhang on all four sides (page ix). Remember to trim the inside to the finished size before adding the second side with overhang.

2 On both of the 19-inch sides, cut slits in the overhang that are even with the edge of the folder and fold in the flaps created.

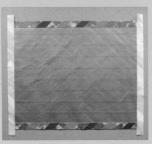

3 Measure, mark, and cut slits in the overhang on both sides at 4 inches and 8 inches up from the folded bottom edge.

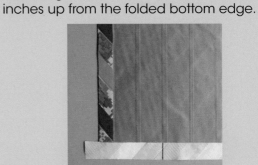

4 Remove the excess overhang from the corners and fold in the flaps that were created above and below the slits.

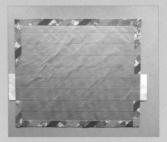

5 Cut slight angles in the corners of the remaining overhang.

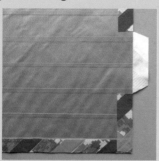

6 Fold up the bottom 4 inches of the folder and secure with the overhang.

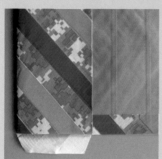

7 Place 1-inch strips of tape on the inside corners of the pocket and fold them over for reinforcement.

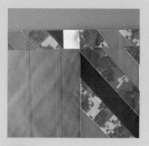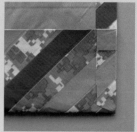

8 Fold the folder in half. To make the folder binder-ready, use another folder or sheet of notebook paper as a template to mark and punch the three holes.

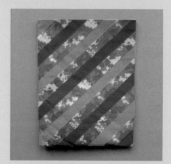

Binder Pouch

Anyone can buy an ordinary pencil case. Make your own and stand out from the crowd.

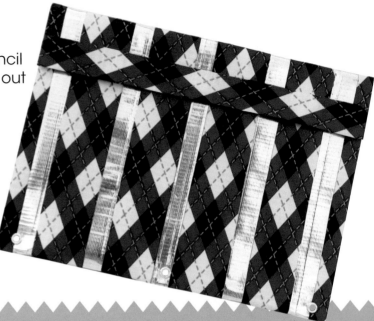

■ ■ ■ ■ ■ ■ ■ ■ ■ ■ ■ ■ ■

ADDITIONAL MATERIALS:
Velcro
Hole punch
Eyelets (optional)

■ ■ ■ ■ ■ ■ ■ ■ ■ ■ ■ ■

1 Make the pouch by creating a 9½ x 16-inch double-sided fabric sheet with overhang on three sides (page x).

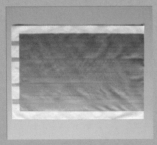

2 Cut slits in the overhang on the end that are even with the corners and fold in the flap created.

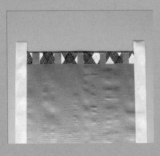

3 Measure 7 inches from the bottom of the folded end and cut slits in the overhang on both sides.

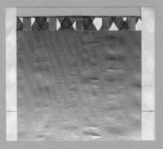

4 Fold in the flaps that are created on the sides of the unfinished end.

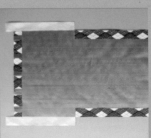

5 Cut angles in the corners of the remaining overhang.

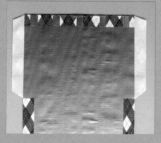

6 Create the pocket by folding the sheet at the 7-inch mark and using the overhang to close the sides.

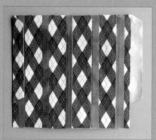

7 Cut an 11½-inch strip of tape to wrap the unfinished end (page xi).

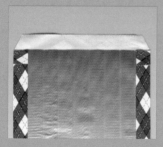

8 Fold over the pouch flap and add Velcro to secure it.

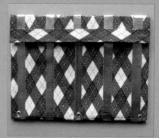

9 Use a sheet of notebook paper as a template to mark where the holes should be and punch them out. Insert eyelets in each hole, if using.

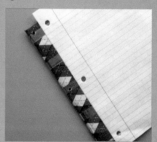

Blooming Pen

Everyone's going to want to use your pen and then want you to make one for them.

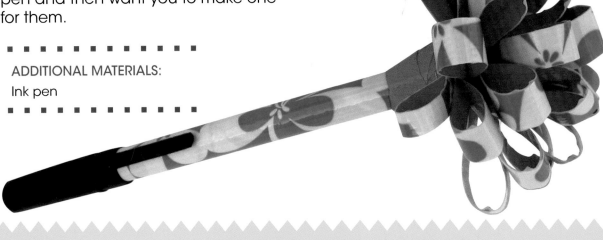

▪ ▪ ▪ ▪ ▪ ▪ ▪ ▪ ▪ ▪ ▪ ▪

ADDITIONAL MATERIALS:

Ink pen

▪ ▪ ▪ ▪ ▪ ▪ ▪ ▪ ▪ ▪ ▪ ▪

1 To cover the pen, cut a strip of tape that is long enough to cover the pen with the cap on.

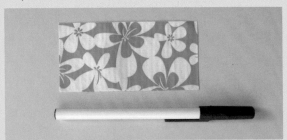

2 Remove the cap and roll the strip of tape around the pen.

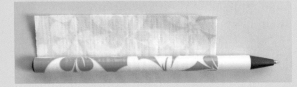

3 To create the petals, cut one 2-inch and one 3-inch strip of tape.

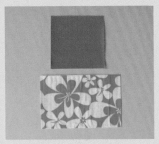

4 Lay the 3-inch strip sticky-side up on the cutting mat and place the 2-inch strip on top of it so that the sticky sides meet. Make it slightly uneven so that there is a little more adhesive on one side.

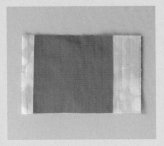

5 Divide the strip into smaller ¼-inch strips.

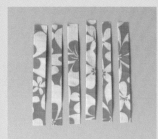

6 Stick one strip across the top of the pen, creating a loop.

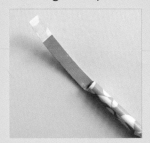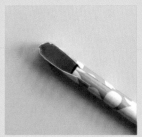

7 Fold the remaining strips in half so that the sticky sides meet, but leave some adhesive exposed.

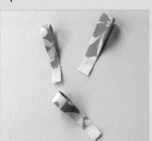

8 Using the sticky side, place the strips around the pen overlapping them slightly. Continue to create and place as many strips as you would like.

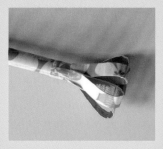

9 Wrap small strips of tape around the bottom of the strips to secure them to the pen.

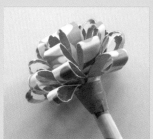

Snack Sack

This snack sack is so alluring that you may eat all of your goodies before reaching your destination.

■ ■ ■ ■ ■ ■ ■ ■ ■ ■ ■ ■ ■

ADDITIONAL MATERIALS:

Velcro

■ ■ ■ ■ ■ ■ ■ ■ ■ ■ ■ ■ ■

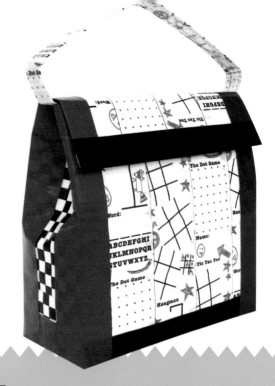

1 To make the pieces, create two double-sided fabric sheets, one that is 10 x 14 inches and another that is 6 x 7 inches (page ix).

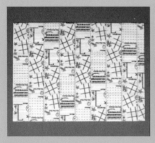

2 Cut the 6 x 7 sheet in half to create two 3 x 7-inch sheets.

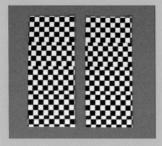

3 Cut two 3-inch strips of tape and trim the top edge of the strips (page xi).

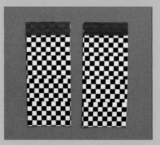

4 Cut the 10 x 14-inch sheet in half lengthwise, and then cut 3 inches off of the top of one of the sheets. This bigger sheet should now be three sheets: one that is 7 x 10 inches, one that is 7 x 7, and another that is 3 x 7.

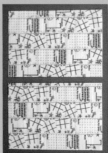
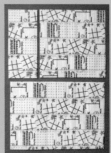

5 Lay the three 3 x 7 sheets wrong-side up on the cutting mat in a row with the ends lined up. Use two 3-inch pieces of tape to connect them. This will create the bottom and sides of the sack.

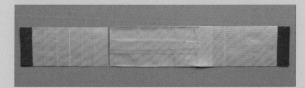

6 Line up the two remaining sheets with the center bottom strip and secure the same way with two 7-inch strips of tape. These will create the front and back of the sack.

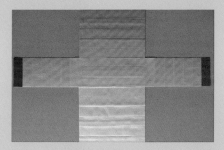

7 Cut four 7-inch strips of tape and place them halfway over the side strips to create overhang.

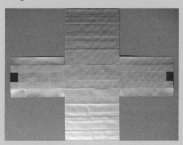

8 Lift one of the sides with overhang and the side next to it, and join them with the overhang to form a corner.

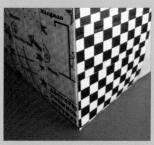

9 Continue with the other corners making sure to firmly press the tape down on the inside.

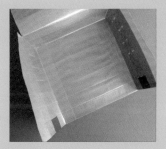

10 Use a 7-inch strip of tape to trim the front edge.

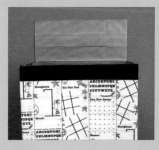

11 Use two 7-inch strips of tape to trim the bottom edges.

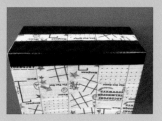

12 Using a 10-inch strip of tape and beginning at the bottom edge of the front side, center the strip halfway over the tote and wrap it around to the top.

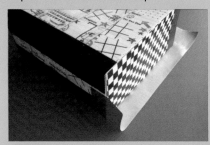

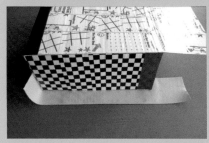

13 Where the side ends, cut an angled slit and fold in the flap.

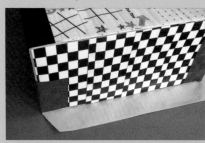

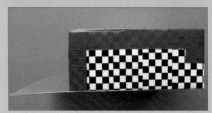

14 Repeat on the other front corner.

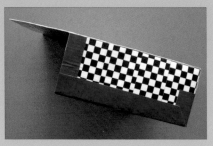

15 Use the same method with two 13-inch strips of tape to cover the back seams. Where the side ends, cut an angled slit and fold in the flap to trim the top edge. Trim off any excess.

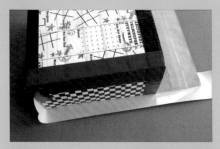

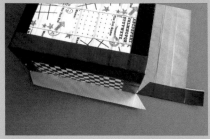

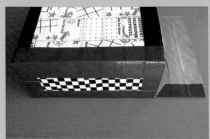

16 Use a 9-inch strip of tape to trim the flap edge (page xi).

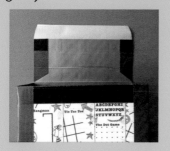

17 To add a handle, create an 18-inch double-layer folded strap (page x).

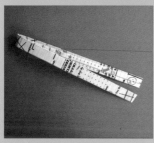

18 Place the strap under the flap where you would like to attach it.

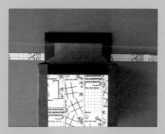

19 Fold the ends to the center and use a small strip of tape to hold them in place.

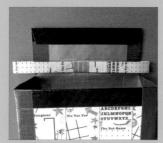

20 Cut a 7-inch strip of tape and use it to secure the handle to the sack.

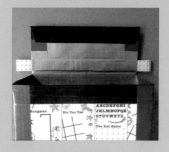

21 Add Velcro to close.

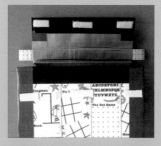

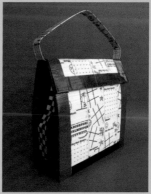

Guy Stuff

Being the mother of all boys, I know how difficult it can be to find craft projects that appeal to them. Here are some projects that are sure to be worthy of their attention and time. However, girls will probably like them, too.

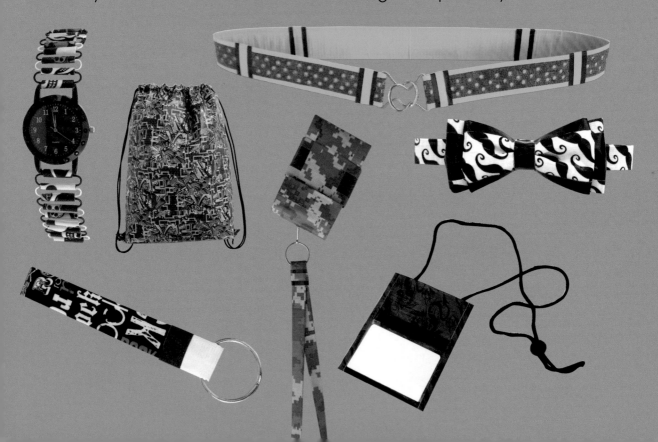

Key Chain

ADDITIONAL MATERIALS:
Split key ring

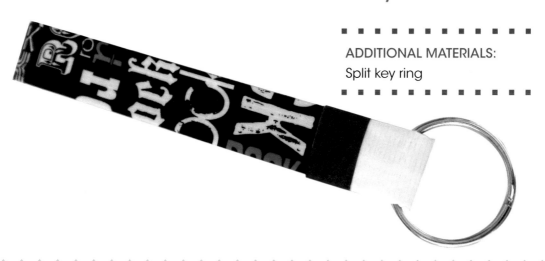

1 Make a 10-inch double layer strap (page x).

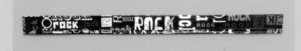

2 Slide the key ring onto the strap.

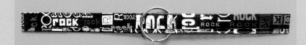

3 With the seam on the inside, bring the ends of the strap together as if you were making a circle. Use a small piece of tape to help hold them in place.

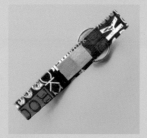
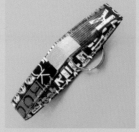

4 Wrap a 3-inch strip of tape around the ends to connect them.

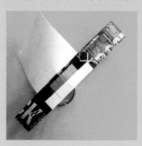
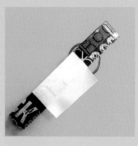

5 Fold the strap in half with the sealed ends facing down and bring the key ring down into the sealed fold.

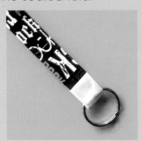

6 Cut a 3 x ½-inch strip of tape and wrap it around the bottom of the key chain to cover the seam.

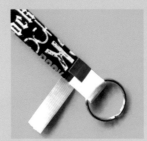
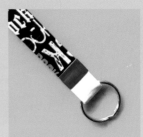

ID Pouch

You'll be able to keep track of your ID, money, ear buds, or other items wearing this super sporty holder.

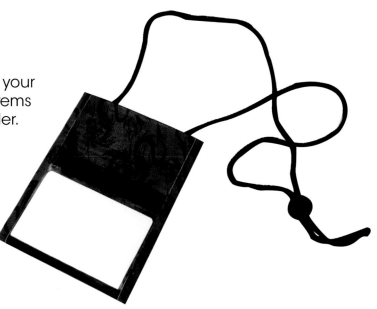

■ ■ ■ ■ ■ ■ ■ ■ ■ ■ ■ ■

ADDITIONAL MATERIALS:

Cording, shoe string, or yarn
Sheet protector or other plastic
Velcro
Hole punch
Eyelets (optional)

■ ■ ■ ■ ■ ■ ■ ■ ■ ■ ■ ■

1 Create a 4 x 10-inch double-sided fabric sheet with overhang on all four sides (page ix) and place it sticky-side down on the mat.

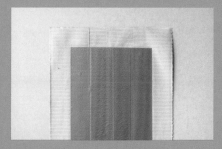

2 Cut a 3 x 4-inch rectangle out of the sheet protector.

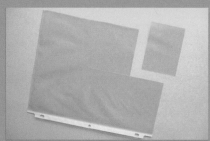

3 Use a 4-inch strip of tape cut in half lengthwise to trim the open edge of the plastic cut-out.

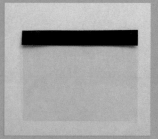

4 Place the plastic cutout on the double-sided sheet 6 inches from the end and 1 inch from either side. Secure it with a 6-inch strip of tape. Measure and make marks if needed.

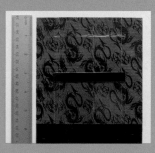

5 Cut a 12-inch strip of tape in half lengthwise and use the strips to secure the edges of the cutout.

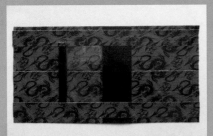

6 Place the pouch sticky-side up. Cut slits at the ends even with the corners and fold in the flaps created.

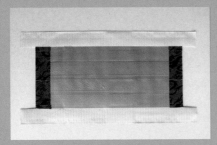

7 Measure, mark, and cut slits on both sides of the overhang at the center. This should be at the bottom of the cutout, 5 inches from both sides of the folded edge.

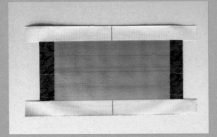

8 On the half of the sheet without the cutout, remove the excess overhang and fold in the flaps on either side.

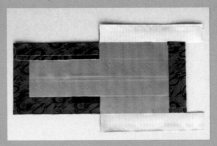

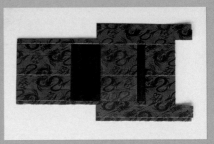

9 Cut slight angles in the remaining overhang.

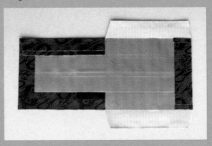

10 Punch two holes in the end without overhang.

11 Fold the pouch in half and secure with the overhang.

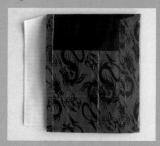

12 Re-punch the holes if needed. Insert eyelets into the holes, if using. Feed the cording through the holes and tie knots in the ends to secure it.

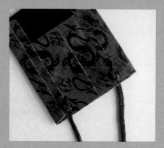

13 Add Velcro to the inside of both the pouch and the ID pocket.

Double Bow Tie

Express your style and be different from the rest in your one-of-a-kind double layered bow tie.

ADDITIONAL MATERIALS:
Velcro

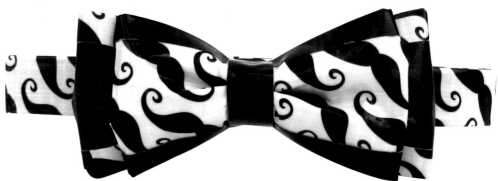

1 Create a 16-inch double-layer folded strap (page x).

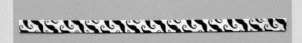

2 Create two double-sided strips that are 9 inches and 7 inches long (page ix).

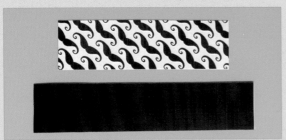

3 Trim each double-sided strip with two additional strips of tape cut in half lengthwise (page ix).

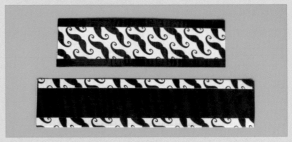

4 Place the two strips wrong-side up on the cutting mat.

5 Fold in the ends of each strip so that they meet in the center. Secure both with pieces of tape that wrap around the edges.

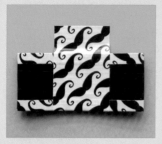

6 Stack the folded strips largest to smallest.

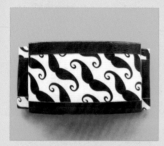

7 Pinch the center to form the bow shape, and wrap the center with a thin strip of tape to retain the shape.

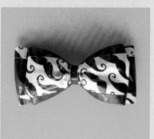

8 Place the bow in the center of the folded strap. Secure them together by wrapping a thin 5-inch strip of tape around the center.

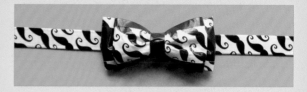

9 A strip of tape can be added across the back as reinforcement.

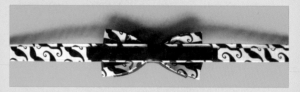

10 Trim the length if needed and wrap the ends (page xi).

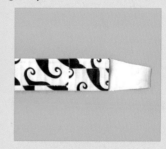

11 Add Velcro to fit.

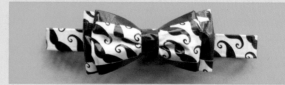

Cell Phone Case with Optional Lanyard

ADDITIONAL MATERIALS:

Velcro
Optional Lanyard Materials:
Hole punch
Eyelets (optional)
Split key ring
Lanyard hook

Your phone will always have a place when you store it in your duct tape case.

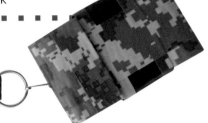

1 Measure and create a double-sided fabric sheet that is at least ¼ inch wider and 3 times longer than your phone (page ix).

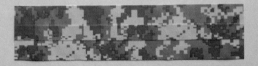

2 Use two strips of tape the same length as the sheet to trim both sides (page xi).

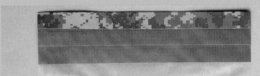

3 Create a double-sided strip long enough to wrap around the short side of the phone (page ix).

4 Trim both sides of the strip (page xi).

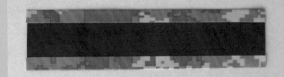

5 Place the phone on the sheet and fold the bottom up to create a pocket.

6 Place the double-sided strip around the sheet with the phone in it. Secure it with a small piece of tape.

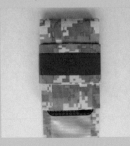
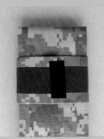

7 Cut a strip of tape the same length as the original double-sided fabric sheet and place it down the center of the sheet to secure the strip.

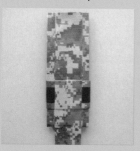 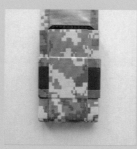

8 With the outer flap of the case pulled back, use a strip of tape to wrap the inside edge of the case to hold down the horizontal strip and finish the ends of the sheet (page xi).

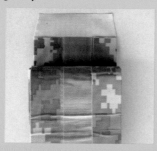

9 Use another strip of tape to wrap the flap end.

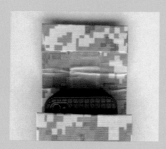

10 Add Velcro to the flap for closure.

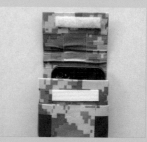

11 To add a lanyard to the case, make two holes in the top center of the flap. Insert eyelets into the holes, if using. Make the lanyard as instructed on page 46.

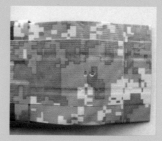

12 Feed the lanyard hook through both of the holes.

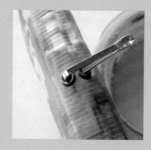 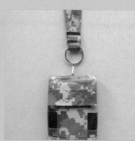

Belt

Design a belt that's as cool as you are.

ADDITIONAL MATERIALS:

Latching belt buckle
Hole punch

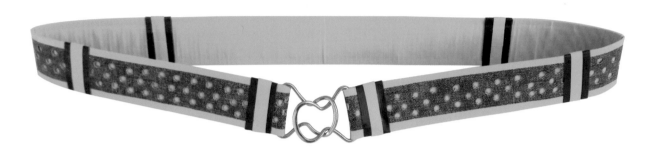

1 Create a double-sided strip that is the same length as your belt or at least 4 inches longer than your waist (page ix).

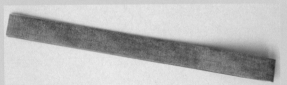

2 It can be difficult to work with a very long strip, so piece short strips together if necessary by overlapping the ends with strips of tape. They can be covered and used as a design later.

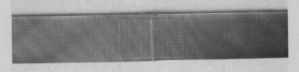

3 Trim the strip to a width of 1¼ inches or slightly smaller than the width of the rings of the belt buckle.

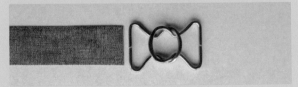

4 Punch holes lengthwise down the center of the strip in any pattern.

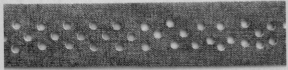

5 Cut a strip of tape the same length as the belt and place it sticky side up on the mat. If several pieces were used, use the same lengths.

6 Cut another strip of the same length in half lengthwise and place it in the center of the sticky strip so that the sticky sides meet.

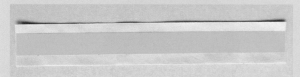

7 Center the belt strip on the sticky strip so that the color shows through the holes.

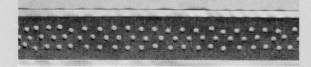

8 Fold down the overhang to trim the belt.

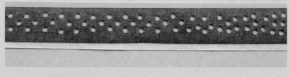

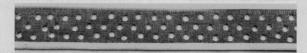

9 Place one end of the belt through a buckle and fold it over about an inch.

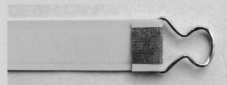

10 Cut a 6-inch strip of tape in half lengthwise and wrap it around the belt to secure the fold.

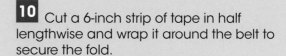

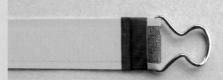

11 Add an accent with an additional strip of tape.

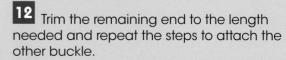

12 Trim the remaining end to the length needed and repeat the steps to attach the other buckle.

13 Use the same size strips with accents to cover the piecing seams and finish the design.

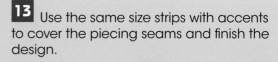

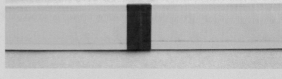

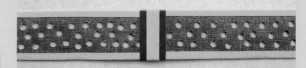

Watch Band Links

Don't throw away your watch just because the band is old and worn. Give it new life with taped paper clip links.

▪ ▪ ▪ ▪ ▪ ▪ ▪ ▪ ▪ ▪ ▪

ADDITIONAL MATERIALS:

Paper clips
Wire cutters
Watch face
Two lobster clasps

▪ ▪ ▪ ▪ ▪ ▪ ▪ ▪ ▪ ▪

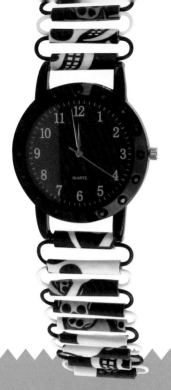

1 Clip the small center loop off of several paper clips.

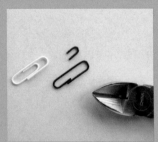

2 Cut several pieces of tape that are slightly narrower than the paper clip.

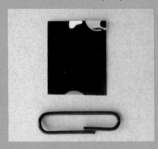

3 Place the flat end of a paper clip against the pin of the watch and wrap a piece of tape around the two to join them together.

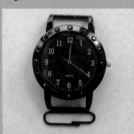
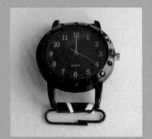

4 Continue adding and wrapping paper clips until they reach halfway around your arm.

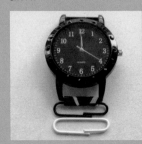
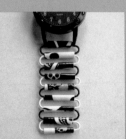

5 Repeat on the other side of the watch.

6 When you get to the last paper clip needed, slide on the lobster clasps and push them toward the ends.

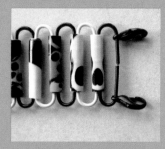

7 Seal the side shut with another piece of tape.

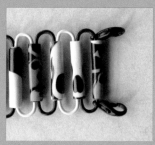

8 Use the clasps to close the watch.

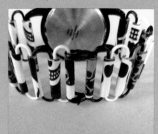

Drawstring Backpack

This bag will be perfect for carrying a few of your things. Show some spirit by making one in your school or team colors.

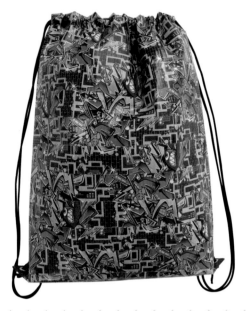

■ ■ ■ ■ ■ ■ ■ ■ ■ ■ ■ ■

ADDITIONAL MATERIALS:

Hole punch
Eyelet (optional)
Two (72-inch) lengths of cording, yarn, or rope
   or a pair of 72-inch shoelaces
Long stick

■ ■ ■ ■ ■ ■ ■ ■ ■ ■ ■ ■

1 Create two 14 x 19-inch double-sided fabric sheets with overhang on one end (page ix).

2 Fold down the sides with overhang 2 inches to create a small opening at the top of the sheets.

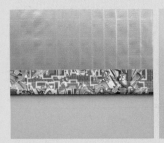
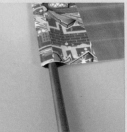

3 Use 14-inch strips of tape to secure the entire width of each overhang. There should be no exposed adhesive in the openings.

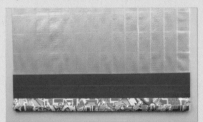

4 Place the bottom ends of the sheets together and secure on both the inside and the outside with 14-inch strips of tape.

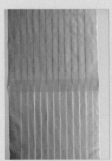

5 Fold the sheets together to close them. Use two 17-inch strips of tape to trim the sides, sealing them shut (page xi). Do not seal the openings of the holes.

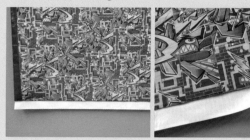

6 Pinch the bottom corners of the bag to create a flat bottom as wide as you would like.

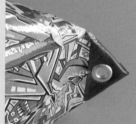

7 Use a small strip of tape to reinforce the corners, then make holes in them. Insert eyelets, if using.

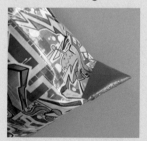

8 Temporarily tape or tie the 72-inch piece of string to the end of the stick.

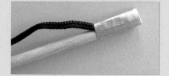

9 Thread the string in through one side of the bag and out through the other side in a clockwise direction. The string should loop around one side of the bag and both ends should end up on the same side of the bag. Remove the stick.

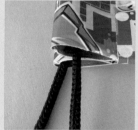

10 Making sure that the ends are even, place them through the bottom hole on the same side and knot them to secure.

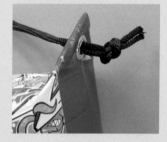

11 Repeat with the other 72-inch piece of string, but thread it through the bag in the opposite, or counterclockwise, direction.

12 Feed the ends through the bottom hole on that side and knot to secure.

13 Pull the strings in opposite directions to create the drawstring effect. The tape will be rigid at first but will become easier to gather as you continue to use the bag.

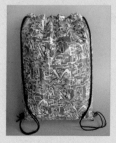

Drawstring Backpack

Party Time

Many budgets are tight these days, resulting in more of us looking for DIY options for party decorating and planning. Here are a few inexpensive ways to add to your party experience. You can even get your guests involved in the duct tape fun by letting them make hats, or key chain or bracelet favors.

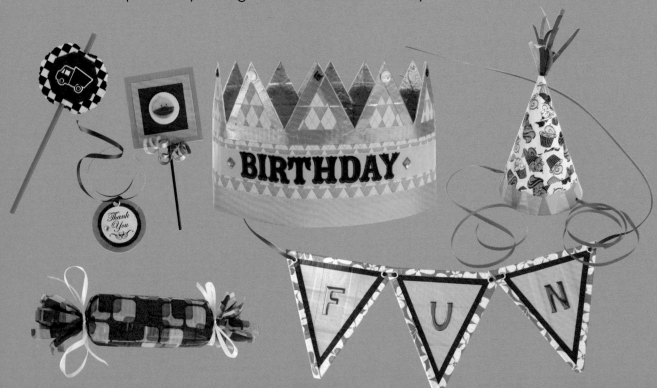

Banner

Surprise! When you design it yourself, you can make a banner for any occasion that says whatever you'd like.

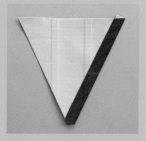

ADDITIONAL MATERIALS:

Ruler
Hole punch
Eyelets (optional)
Ribbon or string
Letter stickers

1 Create a 5-inch square double-sided fabric sheet (page ix).

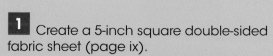

3 Use 6-inch strips of tape cut in half lengthwise to trim all three sides (page xi). Cut off any excess.

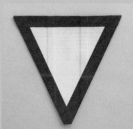

2 Draw a triangle from the bottom corners to the top center of the sheet and cut it out.

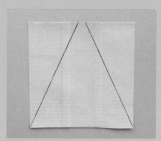

4 Add more trim with three additional 6-inch strips of tape. In order to cover the back, do not cut these in half.

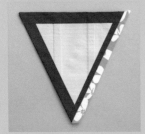 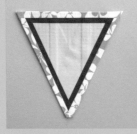

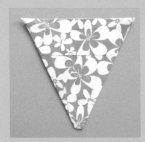

5 Punch holes in the two top corners. Add eyelets, if using.

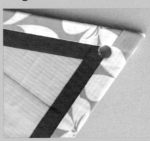

6 Create as many banner pieces as desired and string together for hanging. Use a letter on each piece to spell out your message.

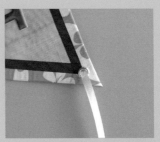

Party Tags

Enhance the theme of your party or leave little messages for your guests. You can attach party tags to items like gifts, lollipop sticks, cocktail and cupcake picks, or straws.

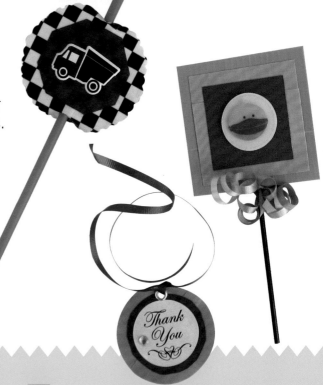

. . . .

ADDITIONAL MATERIALS:

Curling ribbon, straws, or toothpicks
Hole punch

. . . .

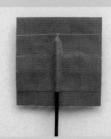

1 Create a double-sided fabric sheet and draw a shape in the desired size (page ix).

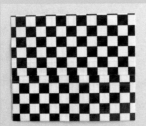

2 Cut out the shapes. Avoid plain edges by using decorative scissors.

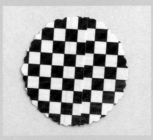

3 To create a layered look with multiple colors, cut out and add slightly smaller shapes.

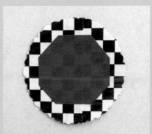

For Toothpicks: Place the pick on the back of the shape and secure with strips of tape. Complete with ribbon.

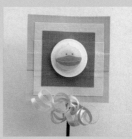

For Straws: Punch holes near the top and bottom of the shape and thread the straw through both.

For Labels: Punch a hole at the top of your shape and string with curling ribbon.

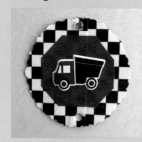 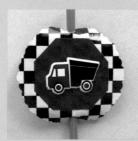 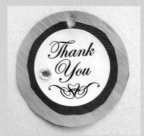 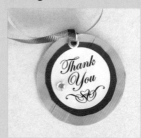

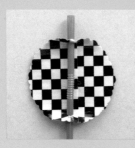

Favor Rolls

With a wrapper this cute, your guests just might forget that there's a treat inside.

■ ■ ■ ■ ■ ■ ■ ■ ■ ■ ■ ■ ■

ADDITIONAL MATERIALS:

Tissue paper
Curling ribbon
Favors

■ ■ ■ ■ ■ ■ ■ ■ ■ ■ ■ ■

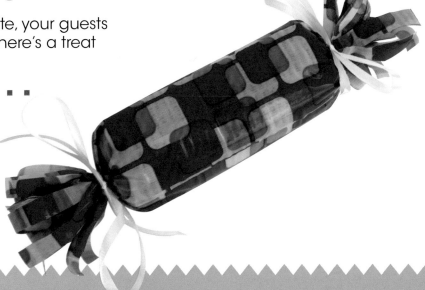

1 Cut a sheet of tissue paper several inches longer than the items being given and wide enough to wrap around them.

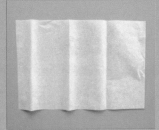

2 Cover one side of the tissue paper with slightly overlapping strips of tape and trim off any excess paper.

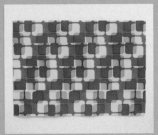

3 Place your items on the tissue side of the sheet and roll it up. Be sure to leave a few inches on either end. Secure with a small piece of tape.

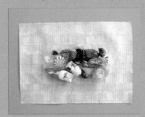 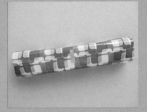

4 Secure with a strip of tape long enough to cover the entire seam.

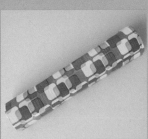

5 Gather the ends, tie them off with pieces of ribbon, and cut slits to create fringe.

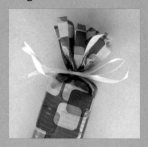 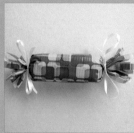

6 Add a little extra something by attaching a party tag (page 77).

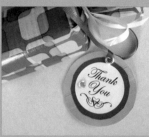

Party Hat

Have each of your guests create their own unique party hat to help celebrate the day.

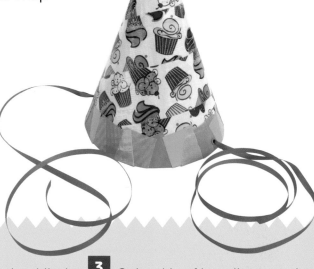

- - - - - - - - - - -

ADDITIONAL MATERIALS:

Party hat template
Curling ribbon

- - - - - - - - - - -

1 Create a double-sided fabric sheet that is the same size as a sheet of paper (page ix).

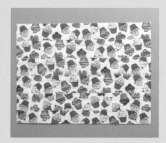

2 Print out a party hat template (search online for one), trace it onto the sheet, and cut it out.

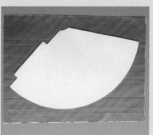

3 Cut a strip of tape the same length as the sides and place it halfway over one edge.

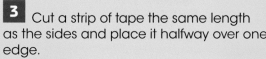

4 Cut several pieces of ribbon and use a small piece of tape to hold them together.

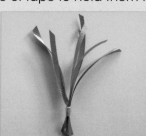

5 Tape the bundle of ribbon to the inside top of the sheet.

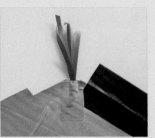

6 Fold the sheet into the hat shape and secure on the inside with the overhang.

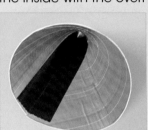

7 Use a strip of tape longer than the hat to cover the outside seam and fold it to the inside.

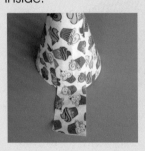 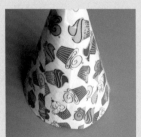

8 Fold 1-inch pieces of tape over the bottom edge of the hat to decorate.

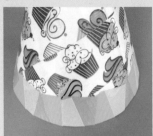

9 Make a hole on either side of the hat and string a piece of ribbon through each.

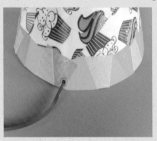

10 Knot and tape down the ends of the ribbons on the inside to secure.

Special Day Crown

Let everyone know it's your day with a personalized crown fit for any prince or princess.

. . . .

ADDITIONAL MATERIALS:

Velcro (optional)

. . . .

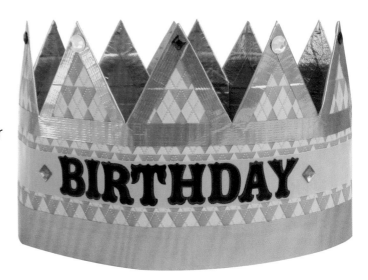

1 Create a double-sided fabric sheet that is 5 inches wide and at least 2 inches longer than your head (page ix).

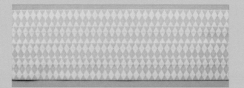

2 On the back side, draw and cut out triangles at the top of the sheet. You can mix things up by making the triangles different sizes.

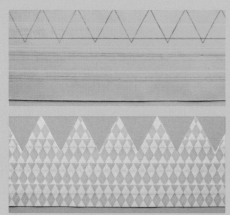

3 Trim the bottom edge with a strip of tape the same length as the sheet (page xi).

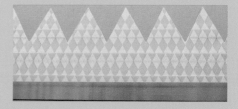

4 Cut strips of tape in half lengthwise and use them to trim the sides of the triangles.

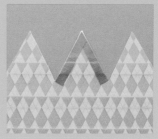

5 Cut additional strips of tape the same length as the sheet to accent.

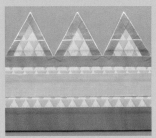

6 To permanently close the crown, place the ends together and cover the seams with a long strip of tape that folds over the bottom edge to the inside.

7 If you want the crown to open or be adjustable, trim the ends and add Velcro.

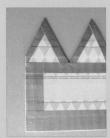

Roll Recycling

Using as much duct tape as I do, I end up with a countless amount of empty rolls. Since I'm also a big fan of recycling whenever possible, I decided to combine the two. After emptying your rolls by creating all of the other cool projects in the book, try these designs.

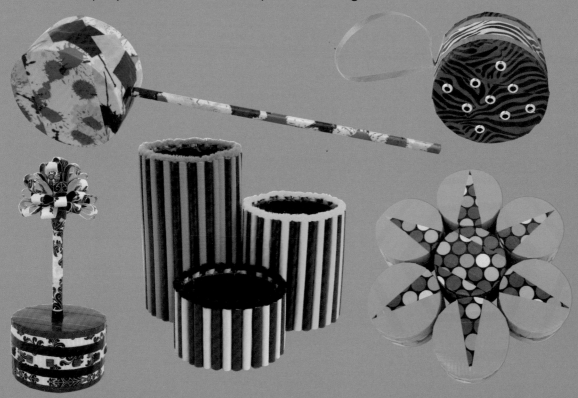

Empty Duct Tape Roll Cover Technique

■ ■ ■ ■ ■ ■ ■ ■ ■ ■ ■

ADDITIONAL MATERIALS:
Cardboard or cardstock

■ ■ ■ ■ ■ ■ ■ ■ ■ ■ ■

1 Make a circle by tracing the outside of an empty roll onto cardstock or cardboard and cutting it out.

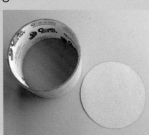

2 Create a 5-inch square single-sided fabric sheet (page ix). Turn it sticky-side up, place the circle in the center, and press down firmly.

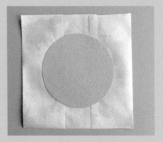

3 Cut slits in the overhang from the cutout to the outer edge around the entire sheet.

4 Place the empty roll on top of the circle and fold over all the strips to secure.

5 Repeat for the other side if necessary.

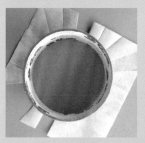

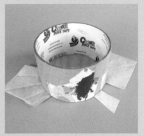

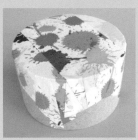

Decorative Air Fresheners

These air fresheners will not only smell great but look fabulous, too!

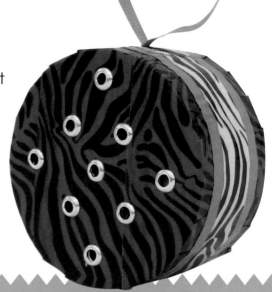

■ ■ ■ ■ ■ ■ ■ ■ ■ ■ ■ ■ ■

ADDITIONAL MATERIALS:

Empty duct tape roll
Potpourri or scent bag
Ribbon or string
Eyelets (optional)

■ ■ ■ ■ ■ ■ ■ ■ ■ ■ ■ ■ ■

For a hanging air freshener:

1 Create two covers for the empty tape roll and poke several holes in them (page 86). Be sure not to make the holes too large or the potpourri will fall out. Insert eyelets into the holes, if desired.

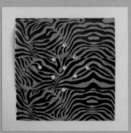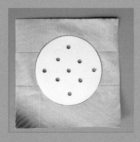

2 Make a small hole in the side of the empty duct tape roll that is large enough to fit the ribbon through.

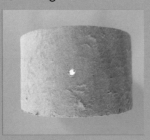

3 Attach one of the covers to the roll (page 86).

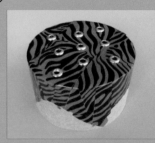

4 With the ribbon folded in half evenly, place the ends through the hole from the outside and tape them down to keep it from sliding back out.

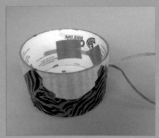

5 Add potpourri to the center of the empty roll.

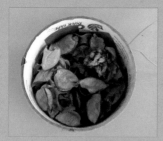

7 Layer 11-inch strips of tape and place them around the outside to finish.

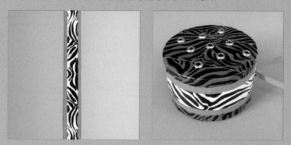

6 Place the other cover on top and secure.

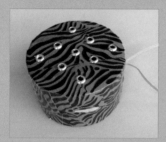

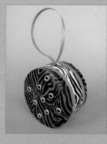

For a tabletop air freshener:

Only poke holes in the top cover and omit the ribbon steps.

Pen Holder

A pen holder would make a great gift for someone's desk. Give one to your mom, dad, and favorite teacher. Just don't forget to include a pen.

■ ■ ■ ■ ■ ■ ■ ■ ■ □ ■ ■ □

ADDITIONAL MATERIALS:

Empty duct tape roll
Styrofoam
Pen
Glue (optional)

■ ■ ■ ■ ■ ■ ■ ■ ■ □ ■ ■ □

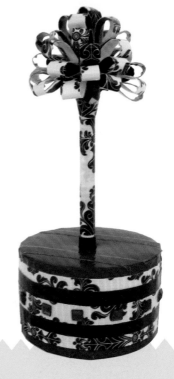

1 Create two covers for the empty tape roll, but only attach one for the bottom (page 86).

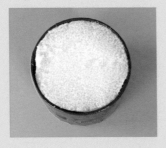

2 Glue a piece of Styrofoam into the empty roll. The Styrofoam does not have to fill the entire space as long as there is some in the center.

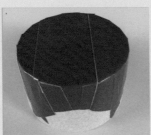

3 Poke a hole slightly larger than the diameter of the pen in the center of the other cover. Attach it to the top of the roll.

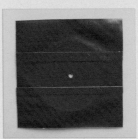 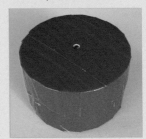

4 Cut and layer several 11-inch strips of tape to wrap around the outside of the holder.

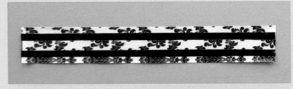

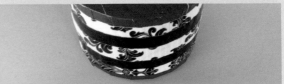

5 If the pen does not have a cap, gently push it into the hole as far as you would like.

6 If it has a cap, use the cap to create the correct size hole. If you don't want the cap to come out when the pen is removed, use a small amount of glue in the hole to secure it in place.

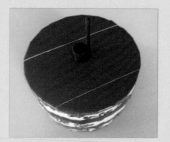

7 Check out the Blooming Pen project to create a unique matching pen and holder set (page 52).

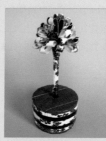

Wall Art

Not being an artist doesn't mean you can't create wonderful works of art. Group together several small wall art clusters and watch your masterpiece appear.

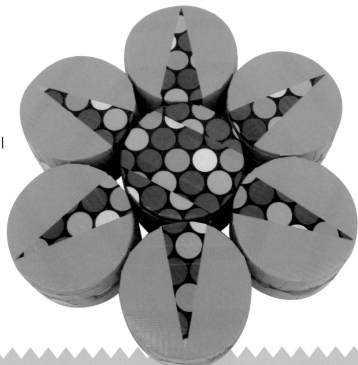

■ ■ ■ ■ ■ ■ ■ ■ ■ ■ ■ ▢

ADDITIONAL MATERIALS:

Empty duct tape roll
Glue for plastic or hot glue gun,
   or small screws with nuts

■ ■ ■ ■ ■ ■ ■ ■ ■ ■ ▢

1 Decide on a pattern and size for your wall art cluster.

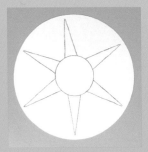

2 Create and attach covers to one side of the empty tape rolls that follow the pattern.

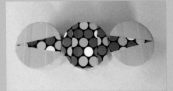

3 Cover the outside and bottom edge of the rolls with 3-inch strips of tape overlapped and folded to the inside.

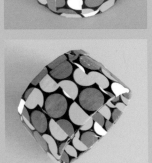

4 Arrange the pattern and glue the sides of the rolls that touch together.

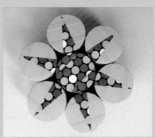

5 For a more secure hold, make holes on the inside and attach the rolls with small screws and nuts.

6 Since the back side is open, you can hang the cluster on the wall with nails.

Maracas

If you're having a party or attending an event where noise making is expected, then make plenty of it with this unexpected noise maker.

■ ■ ■ ■ ■ ■ ■ ■ ■ ■ ■ ■

ADDITIONAL MATERIALS:

Empty duct tape roll
Wooden dowel
Uncooked small pasta or rice
Glue

■ ■ ■ ■ ■ ■ ■ ■ ■ ■ ■

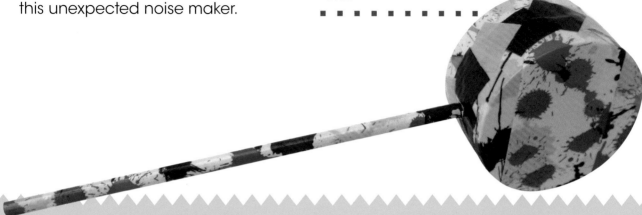

1 Make a hole in the side of the empty duct tape roll that is large enough to fit the dowel through.

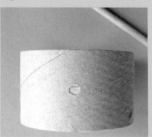

2 Slide the dowel through the hole until it reaches the top of the inside of the roll. Make a mark around the dowel where the roll ends.

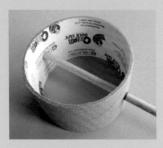

3 Remove the dowel from the hole. Use the mark to measure and cut a strip of tape that is long enough to cover the dowel from the mark to the bottom end.

4 Wrap the strip of tape around the dowel.

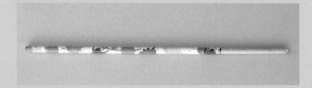

5 Create two covers for the empty tape roll but only attach one (page 86).

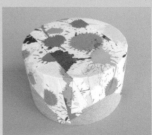

6 Insert the dowel back into the empty roll. Add glue to the top of the dowel and the inside of the roll where they will meet to secure them together. Allow the glue to dry. (Pieces of tape can also be used to secure the dowel.)

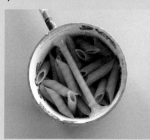

7 Fill the center of the roll halfway with the uncooked pasta or rice.

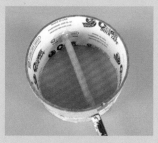

8 Attach the other cover to the open side.

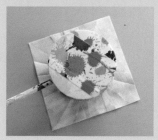

9 Cut 1-inch squares of tape and place them randomly around the outside to decorate.

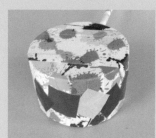

Desk Organizers

These containers allow you to be organized and stylish at the same time. Perfect for desk items like paper clips, crayons, pencils, and scissors, or any other items that often get lost at the bottom of a drawer.

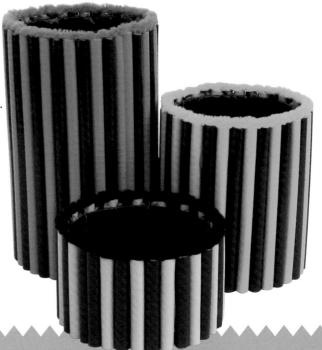

ADDITIONAL MATERIALS:

Empty duct tape rolls
Drinking straws
Pipe cleaners
Glue for plastic or hot glue gun

1 Create and attach a cover to one side of an empty tape roll to form the bottom (page 86).

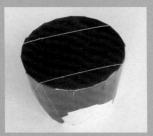

2 Cover the inside and the rim of the roll with 3-inch strips of tape by placing them against the inside bottom and folding them over the outer edge. The strips can be cut in half lengthwise to make them easier to work with.

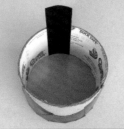 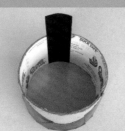

3 Overlap the strips slightly all the way around.
Note: Covering the inside and rim is optional. It's up to you if you would like the duct tape logo to show.

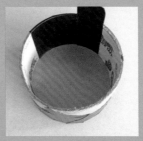 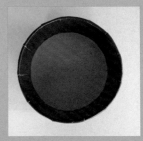

4 Cut a strip of tape longer than the height of the roll and wrap it around the straw.

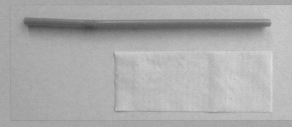

5 Add a line of glue to the outside of the empty tape roll or the straw and place the straw vertically onto the roll.

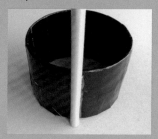

6 Continue gluing straws until the entire tape roll is covered. Trim the excess straw as you go.

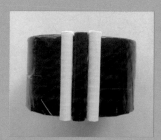

7 Decorate the top of the organizer by cutting pipe cleaners in half and placing the ends in every other straw hole.

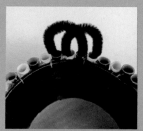 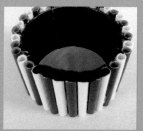

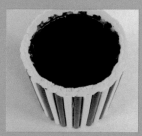

8 To create taller organizers, stack empty tape rolls in groups of two and three and place strips of tape around the seams to connect them.

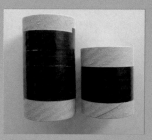

9 Repeat the same steps, adjusting the length of your tape-wrapped straws as needed.

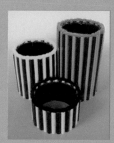

Duct Tape Resources

The following brands of tape were used to create the projects in this book:

Platypus Designer Duct Tape (www.designerducttape.com)
Scotch Brand Duct Tape (www.scotchbrand.com)
ShurTech Brand Duck Tape (www.shurtech.com)

Most of the tools used in this book can be found at craft stores, including:

A.C. Moore (www.acmoore.com)
Hobby Lobby (www.hobbylobby.com)
Jo-Ann Fabric and Craft Stores (www.joann.com)
Michaels (www.michaels.com)

About the Author

Tamara Boykins, an event planner, has been an avid crafter for the past eighteen years. She is committed to fostering creativity and imagination in children through arts and crafts. As a hobby, she has instructed craft classes at parties and community centers that include lessons in one of her favorite mediums, duct tape. She has traveled throughout South Florida selling her duct tape creations at art shows and craft fairs. Her duct tape designs have been featured in the Style section of the *New York Times* and many blogs. Her designs can be found at www.dbyt4u.com. Tamara is a military spouse and the mother of four who resides in Pembroke Pines, Florida.